PEDIATRIC
RADIOLOGICAL SIGNS

PEDIATRIC RADIOLOGICAL SIGNS

Volume II

MICHAEL GRUNEBAUM, M.D.
SPECIALIST IN DIAGNOSTIC RADIOLOGY
AND PEDIATRIC RADIOLOGIST

FORMER RADIOLOGIST-IN-CHIEF,
THE SCHNEIDER CHILDRENS M.C. OF ISRAEL,
THE RABIN CAMPUS,PETACH-TIQVA;
CLINICAL PROFESSOR OF DIAGNOSTIC RADIOLOGY (Emeritus),
SACKLER SCHOOL OF MEDICINE, TEL-AVIV UNIVERSITY, ISRAEL.

iUniverse, Inc.
New York Lincoln Shanghai

PEDIATRIC RADIOLOGICAL SIGNS
Volume II

iUniverse books may be ordered through booksellers or by contacting:

iUniverse
2021 Pine Lake Road, Suite 100
Lincoln, NE 68512
www.iuniverse.com
1-800-Authors (1-800-288-4677)

ISBN-13: 978-0-595-34446-8 (pbk)
ISBN-13: 978-0-595-79206-1 (ebk)
ISBN-10: 0-595-34446-1 (pbk)
ISBN-10: 0-595-79206-5 (ebk)

Printed in the United States of America

Dedicated to—
My grandchildren, Maytav and Eden, Or and Schir and to the twins
Ruth and Yonatan.

And to—
The children around the world for a better health-care and better services.

From all I acquired knowledge: From my mentors, scholars, students, and residents, but above all—from analyzing my own professional msitakes.

(M.G.)

Content

Preface

Now-a-days, at the beginning of the thired melenium, while we have at hand sofistikated imaging modalities, the question comes up wether there is still need of the traditional radiology pediatric radiology?, the definite answer is—**YES** !

There is no simple, efficient, economic and quick substitute other than a radiogram to diagnose pneumonia, bone trauma or identify an intestinal obstruction. All other imaging modalities are of the "second and third line category". Thus, the time has not yet arrived to out-date the analysis of the X-ray film.

The purpose of this book is to give the imaging-physician or the pediatrician (whatever his **subspecialty** might be) a guid-line to match a radiological sign with a suspected clinical entitiy.

The present book is arranged according to the body systems. The list of tables serves as a "road-map" to direct the reader to the "location" of his search. At the beginning of every chapter are grouped those radiological signs dealing with the newborn (pre-term or term infant). The heading of each table includes a joint X-ray sign for various diseases that are arranged in an alphabetical order and not according to their frequency of appearance. This approach was taken by the author as there is a difference in the frequency of the diseases in the various countries around the globe. Adjacent to most of the disease entities is a short explanation, description or hint of the disease itself.

The tables are a collection of the daily work and experience in pediatric radiology gathered over 35 years, as well as from reading textbooks, journals and lectures. The author did not see any use in adding a long list of references that are already quoted in the textbooks to which he refer. A list of recent papers, from various imaging journals (published during the last 4 years) are quoted.

No doubt that this book does not encompass all the situations, signs and existing radiological combinations. Thus, every reader should feel free to add from his own experience and reading, "And the more—the better".

I should like to extend my thanks to Mrs A. Hoepker and Mr J.D. McWilliams from the Publishing House iUniverse, in guiding and helping me to publish this book.

(M.G., March 2004)

The list of tables

Chapter 15: The urinary tract
Newborn:

Infancy and childhood:
The kidney

Chapter 16: The Adrenal Gland

Chapter 17: The Retroperitoneal Space

Chapter 18: The Male Genital Organs

Chapter 19: The Female Genital Organs

Chapter 20: References

Chapter 21: Index of the Various Iimaging Signs

Chapter 11

The Biliary System

(The examination of choice of the bile duct system is—ultrasonography completed or started with a plain abdominal film)

1. Neonatal obstructive jaundice
Alpha-1- antitrypsin deficiency
Biliary abnormalities:
    Choledochal cyst (Choledochocoele. A dilatation of the intramural portion of the distal common bile duct within the duodenal wall)
    Hypoplasia
    Inspisated bile p;ug syndrome
Obstruction
Cholestasis due to total parenteral nutrition
Cystic fibrosis (Mucoviscidosis...A multisystem disease characterized by mucus plugging of exocrine glands secondary to a thick tenacious materisl and reduced mucociliary transport)
Galactosemia
Hereditary tyrosinemia
Hyperalimentation (Forming obstructing stones)
Infection:
    Bacterial
    Viral
Neonatal hepatitis

Reference: 18, 26, 36, 45, 66, 111, 118, 120, 123, 131

2. *Gallstones*
After valve replacement
Agh deficiency
Bile ducts anomalies
Chemotherapeutic drugs
Congenital hemolytic anemias
Cystic fibrosis (Mucoviscidosis. A multisystem disease characterized by mucus plugging of exocrine glands secondary to a thick tenacious materisl and reduced mucociliary transport)
Diuretic drugs (Especialy in premature newborns)
Overweight
Parenteral hyperalimentation over a long period
Wilson disease (A metabolic disorder of copper metabolism. Hepatolenticular degeneratin)

Reference: 18, 36, 44, 45, 66, 111, 118, 120, 123, 131
(See also Chapter 15, Table 2)

3. *Gas in the bilary tract*
After Kasai operation
After passage of a billiary stone
After trauma
Emphysematous cholecystitis

Reference: 26, 36, 45, 111, 118

Chapter 12

The Spleen

1. *Splenomegaly (General overview)*
(Nowadays the examination of choice of the spleen is ultrasonography. The plain abdominal film completes the information not detected by the transducer)

Anemias (Aquired or congenital)
Bacterial infection
Burkitt lymphoma (A non-Hodgkin lymphoma, associated with the Epstein-Barr virus and abdominal involvement)
Cirrhosis (Various etiologies associated with ascites)
Collagen disease (Various etiologies)
Congestive heart failure (Associated with cardiac disease and back pressure into the inferior vena cava)
Cystic fibrosis (Due to portal hypertension)
Dermoid cyst in the spleen (Solitary, unilocular, with calcifications)
Echinococcus cyst (Curvilinear or polycyclic calcifications)
Gaucher disease (A cerebroside lipidosis. Due to repeated infarctions)
Granulomatous disease of childhood
Hemangioma (Smal calcification/s. Phlebolith/s)
Hematoma (Trauma causing hemorrhage)
Hemochromatosis (Iron deposition in the parennchymal cells. Due to hemolysis or repeated blood transfusions)
Hemoglobinopathies (Due to active proliferation of the red blood cells)
Hemolitic anemia (Active proliferation of the red blood cells)
Hepatitis (Various etiologies. If leading to portal hypertension than splenomegaly may appear)
Hereditary sphrocytosis (A congenital hemolytic anemia)
Hogkin disease (Infiltrative or wide-spread nodular involvement of the spleen)
Infectious mononucleosis
Langerhans cell histiocytosis

Leukemia (Diffuse leukemic infiltrations throughout the spleen)
Lymphoma (A homogeneous, diffuse infiltration of the spleen)
Malaria
Niemann-Pick disease (A sphingomyelin lipidosis)
Non-Hodgkin lymphoma (Diffuse infiltration of the spleen)
Parasites (Ssplenomegaly with or without calcifications)
Portal hypertension (Various etiologies)
Schistosomiasis (Bilharziasis. Schistozoma haematobium)
Splenic cyst (Congenital cyst. Unilocular)
Splenic infarction (In sickle cell crisis or Gaucher disease)
Splenic vein thrombosis (Splenomegaly with an elongated calcification. Sometimes ascites may be present)
Subacute bacterial endocarditis
Thrombotic thrombocytopenic purpura
Trauma (Subcapsular or parenchymal hemorrhage)
Typhoid fever
Viral disease

Reference: 18, 26, 36, 45, 66, 95, 101, 111, 118, 120, 123, 130, 131

2. *Asplenia syndrome*
(See also Chapter 8, Table 66)

3. *Polysplenia syndrome*
(See also Chapter 8, Table 67)

4. *Splenic calcifications*
Congenital cyst (Unilocular)
Dermoid cyst—Epidermoid (Solitary, unilocular, sometimes with calcifications)
Echinoccocus cyst (Curvilinear or polycyclic calcifications)
Granuloma (Single or multiple calcifications throughout the spleen):
    Brucellosis
    Histoplasmosis
    Tuberculosis
Hematoma (Healed)
Infarction:
    Embolic bacterial endocarditis
    Gauche disease

Obstruction to blood flow in the splenic artery
  Sickle cell disease
Phlebolith/s
Post-traumatic cyst
Pyogenic abscess (Healed)
Vascular calcifications

Reference: 18, 26, 45, 66, 111, 118, 123, 131
(See also Chapter 15, Table 2)

Chapter 13

The Pancreas

(The examination of choic of the retroperitoneal pancreas is the ultrasonographic examination; The plain abdominal film adds complemantary information about the intestinal loops in the vicinity of the organ and additional information about other intraabdominal changes not well appreciated on the ultrasonographic examination)

1. Mass within the pancreas in children
Abscess
Acute pancreatitis
Bleeding-Hematoma
Insulinoma
Lymphoma
Metastasis/es
Pseudocyst

Reference: 18, 26, 36, 45, 66, 68, 95, 101, 111, 118, 120, 123, 131
(See also Chapter 17, Table 1)

2. Mass in the pancreatic tail region in children
Cyst or psudocyst (Post pancreatitis)
Intrathoracic tumor (Overlapping tumor from the lower chest region)
Left adrenal tumor (Displacing or infiltrating the pancreatic tail)
Left perirenal space occupying lesion (Displacing or infiltrating the pancreatic tail)
Left renal tumor (Displacing or infiltrating the pancreatic tail)
Pancreatitis (Inflammatory process in the pancreatic tissue)
Splenic tumor (Overlapping the pancreatic tail)

Reference: 18, 36, 66, 111, 118, 123

3. *Pseudocyst of the pancreas in children*
After pancreatitis
Battered child syndrome (Post hemorrhage)
Drugs (Steroids)
Hereditary pancreatitis
Obstruction of: pancreatic duct
Post infection:
  Hepatitis
  Mumps
Trauma (Vehicle accident)

Reference: 18, 26, 45, 68, 95, 101, 111, 118, 120, 123, 131

4. *Pancreatic calcifications in children*
Chronic pancreatitis (Calcifications throughout the pancreatic tissue or duct)
Cystic fibrosis
Hemangioma
Kwashiokor (Calcifications throughout the pancreatic tissue)
Lymphangioma
Metastasis
Old hematoma

Reference: 18, 26, 45, 66, 111, 118, 120, 123, 131
(See also Chapter 17, Table 5)

Chapter 14

The Peritoneal Cavity

1. Ascites in the newborn *

Bile leakage (Obstruction or perforation in the biliary system)
Chylous ascites (In thoracic duct anomalies or rupture)
Cyst rupture within the abdominal cavity (Various entities)
Hydrometrocolpos (A complication of...)
Hydrops fetalis (Erythroblastosis fetalis)
Idiopathic
Inflammatory process:
    Appendicitis
    Meckel diverticulum
Lymphangiectasia (A congenital malformation of the lymphatic system)
Perforation of a hollow viscus (As in necrotizing enterocoloitis)
Post-abdominal surgery
Rupture of an ovarian cyst
Trauma
Urinary tract:
    Bladder rupture
    Neurogenic bladder (In the "atonic type" of the lower motor neuron lesion)
    Posterior urethral valves
    Urereteral obstruction—Uretero-pelvic
                     Uretero-vesical

Reference: 18, 26, 27, 45, 66, 111, 118, 120, 123, 131
(See also Chapter 9, Table 27)
* Nowadays the examination of choice is abdominal ultrasonography

2. *Pneumoperitoneum in the newborn period*
Abdominal trauma (Various etiologies)
Congenital gastrointestinal muscular wall defect with perforation
Disection from a pneumomediastinum
Duodenal atresia with perforation
Gas forming peritonitis
Imperforate anus with perforation
Ileal atresia with perforation
Leaking from a surgical anastomosis
Meconium ileus with perforation
Necrotizing enterocolitis with perforation
Peforated appendix
Perforated cecum (Hirschsprung disease)
Perforation of a foreign body (Various etiologies)
Post-abdominal surgery
Rupture of an abscess

Reference: 15, 18, 26, 27, 36, 44, 45, 66, 111, 118, 120, 123, 130, 131
(See also Chapter 9, Table 25)

3. *Intraperitoneal calcifications in the newborn*
Intra-abdominal cyst (Various entities)
Meconium peritonitis (A sterile chemical peritonitis caused by perforation of an intestinal obstruction. Small flacksof calcifications scattered throughout the peritoneal cavity)
Post infection:
    Bacterial
    Viral
Vascular calcifications

Reference: 18, 26, 45, 111, 118, 123

4. *Ascites in children* *
Budd-Chiari syndrome (Segmental obstruction of the hepatic venous outflow)
Chronic renal failure (Various etiologies)
Chirrhosis (Various entities)
Congestive heart failure (Right heart failure. Various etiologies)
Constrictive pericarditis (Compresison-constriction of the inferior vena cava)
Hypoproteinemia:

Malabsorption
Protein-loosing enteropathy
Metastasis to the peritoneum
Pancreatitis (The acute form)
Primary intraperitoneal malignancy
Trauma

Reference: 18, 26, 44, 45, 66, 68, 95, 101, 111, 118, 120, 123, 131
(See also Chapter 9, Table 99)
* Nowadays the examination of choice is abdominal ultrasonography

5. *Intraperitoneal space occupying lesion/s in children* *
Abscess
Choledochal cyst (Congenital anomaly)
Intestinal duplication (Congenital anomaly)
Lymphangioma (Congenital anomaly)
Mesenteric cyst (Congenital anomaly)
Mesenteric lymphoma
Omental cyst (Congenital anomaly)
Ovarian cyst (Congenital anomaly)
Pancreatic pseudocyst (Post-inflammatory process penetrating into the peritoneal cavity.)
Renal tumor/s (Various entities)
Ventriculo-peritoneal shunt (Pseudocyst)

Reference: 18, 26, 45, 66, 71, 111, 118, 120, 123, 131
(See also Chapter 9, Table 100)
* Nowadays the examination of choice is abdominal ultrasonography

6. *Intraperitoneal calcifications in children* *
Appendecolith (A laminated calcified concrement in the right lower abdominal quadrant)
Bezoar (Concretions of foreign matter composed of accumulated ingested material in the gastro-intestinal tract)
Calcified thrombus
Hydatid cyst (Calcification/s in the cyst wall)
Infarction of appendices epiploicae (After torsion, thrombosis of the appendices epiploic or due to an inflammation in an adjacent organ such as the appendix or in diverticulosis)
Lymph nodes:

Chronic granulomatous disese
Chronic inflammatory disease
Histoplasmosis
Tuberculosis
Meconium peritonitis (A sterile chemical peritonitis. Small flacks of calcifications scattered throughout the peritoneal cavity)
Mesenteric cyst (After bleeding into the cyst)
Phlebolith/s
Stone in a Meckel diverticulum (Calcification in the right lower abdomen)

Reference: 18, 26, 44, 45, 66, 111, 118, 120, 123, 131, 149a-b
(See also Chapter 9, Table 101)

7. Abnormal intra-abdominal air location in children
Absces (Gas forming agents):
  Hepatic
  Lesser sac
  Kidney
  Liver
Pancreas
  Subphrenic
Chilaiditi syndrome
Gas in the biliary system (Various etiologies)
Inguinal hernia
Perforation:
  Ascending colon
  Cecum
  Endoscopic procedure
  Inflammatory bowel disease (Various entities)
  Rectum
  Stomach
Pneumoperitoneum (Varioue entities)
Pneumoretroperitoneum:
  Dissecting mediastinal air
  Gas formig agents in the urinary tract
  Traumatic rupture of duodenum

Reference: 15, 18, 44, 66, 120, 123, 131
(See also Chapter 9, Tables 88, 89)

8. *Pneumoperitoneum in children*
Blunt abdominal trauma
Disection from pneumomediastinum
Enema tip injury
Foreign body
Gas forming peritonitis
Gastric/intestinal muscular wall defect (Congenital anomaly)
Hirschsprung disease (Perforation at the cecum)
Imperforate anus
Laparoscopy-endoscopy-rectoscopy
Meconium ileus (Due to perforation proximal to the obstruction)
Necrotizing enterocoliitis (Perforation at the site of the necrotic bowel wall)
Pneumatosis intestinalis (Rupture of a gas filled cyst located in the intestinal wall)
Post-abdominal surgery
Rupture of appendix
Rupture of intraperitoneal abscess with gas forming agents
Surgical anastomosis
Toxic megacolon (As acomplication of inflammatory bowel disese):
    Crohn disease
    Ischemic colitis
    Psedomembraneous colitis
    Salmonellosis
    Ulcerative colitis

Reference:21
(See also Chapter 9, Table 95)

9. *Benign Pneumatosis in children*
(See also Chapter 9, Table 96)

Chapter 15

The urinary tract

(Nowadays the examination of choice is ultrasonography completed by a plain abdominal radiogram, voiding urtherocytogram or an intravenous pyelography)

1. *Neonatal abdominal mass/es (General overview)*
Renal and urinary mass lesion/s:
Benign cystic hamartoma (May be associated with tuberous sclerosis. An extrarenal tumor with a lucency on the plain abdominal film)
Bilateral, double collecting system
Bladder distention (Various etiologies)
Fanconi anemia
Horseshoe kidney (A congenital anomaly. The two kidneys are joined by their lower poles through a parenchymal or fibrous isthmus)
Hydronephrosis of the congenital type:
    Ectopic ureterocele (Of the obstructive type)
    Posterior urethral valves
    Prune belly syndrome (Eagle Barrett syndrome. Absent or hypoplastic abdominal wall musculature distended ureters with marked hydronephrosis and undescended testes)
    Severe vesico-ureteral reflux—Bladder neck obstruction
                              Urethral obstruction
    Uretero-pelvic junction obstruction
    Uretero-vesical obstruction
Mesoblastic nephroma (Fetal renal hamartoma. A non-calcified renal mass distorting the collecting system. Does not penetrate into the renal pelvis)
Multicystic dysplastic kidney (A unilateral abdominal mass with a lobulated contour)
Nephroblastoma (Multilocular cystic nephroma. A unilateral-uinifocal well cicumscribed mass with calcifications in its periphery. The mass penetrates into the renal pelvis)
Polycystic kidneys (Infantile type. Bilateral renal enlargement with fetal lobulation)

Renal ectopia:

Crossed ectopia (The distal urteter inserts into the trigone on the side of its normal origin)—Fussed

Separated

Longitudinal ectopia—Intrathoracic

Pelvic

Renal fusion—Horseshoe kidney (See above)

Puncake kidney

Renal malrotation (The collecting system is positioned ventrally with an extrarenal pelvis and ectatic calices)

Renal vein thrombosis (Hematuria. Appearance of an enlarged kidney with a smooth border) may be triggered by:

Birth trauma

Dehydration

Diarrhea

Enterocolitis

Infant of diabetic mother

Left adrenal hemorrhage

Polycythemia

Prematurity

Sepsis

Urinoma (A perirenal pseudocyst due to a tear in a the functioning collecting system):

Bladder outlet obstruction

Calculus obstruction in the collecting systen

Penetrating trauma

Ureteral obstruction with back pressure

Wilms tumor (Nephroblastoma. A palpable mass with hematuria. Compresses renal tissue, distorts the renal calyces and the renal pelvis. Calcifications may be appeare. May cross midline and invade the inferior vena cava)

Non-renal retroperitoneal mass/es:

Abscess

Adrenal hemorrhage(A suprarenal mass displacing the renal):

Birth trauma

Hemorrhagic disorders

Hypoxia

Infant of diabetic mother

Septicemia (Meningococcal septicemia)

Ganglioneuroma (May represent the end-stage of maturation of a neuroblastoma or a benign neoplastic growth of the adrenal gland with calcifications)

Lymphangioma
Neuroblastoma (A suprarenal mass with stippled calcifications. Displacement of the kidney in an inferolateral direction without distorsion of the collecting system. Retroperitoneal extension. Liver and bone metastasis)
Teratoma (Punctate or spiculated calcifications which may resemble bone, associated with a soft-tissue mass in the pelvis)
Genital mass/es:
Hydrocolpos and/or hydro-metro-colpos (Accumulation of fluid within an obstructed uterus and/or vagina):
    Cloacal malformation (Single perineal orifice for the urinary bladder, vagina and rectum)
    Imperforate hymen
    Mayer-Rokitansky-Kuestner-Hauser syndrome (Uterus and vaginal agenesis with an intralabial mass. Abdominal pain and primary amenorrhea)
    Persistent urogenital sinus
    Segmental vaginal atresia
Ovarian cyst
Gastrointestinal mass/es:
Cystic ileal dilatation proximal to atresia (A palpable mass presented with meconium)
Duplication cyst (An abdominal mass located at the mesenteric side of the alimentary canal. The cyst paralells the long axis of the bowel lumen)
Intussusception (Invagination of a proximal intestinal segment [Intussusception] into the leumen of the adjacent dista intestine [Intussuscepiens])
Malrotation with/without volvulus (The duodeno-jejumal junction [The ligament of Treitz] is located lower than the duodenal bulbe and shifted to the right. The cecum is not located in the right lower abdominal quadrant)
Mesothelial cyst (Omental or mesenteric cyst. A uni-locular thin wall cyst. May compress or displace the intestinal loops)
Hepato-spleno-biliary masses:
Cholecystitis (A tender palpable soft-tissue mass in the right upper abdomen)
Choledochal cyst (Obstructive jaundice. A right upper quadrant or a upper mid-abdomen soft-tissue density with displacement of the descending segment of the duodenal loop)
Hemangioendothelioma (Infantile hepatic hemangioma. Hepatomegaly with smal calcificatins)
Hepatomegaly and spelnomegaly (Verious etiologies)
Hydrops of gallblader (A tender palpable mass below the lower liver margin. A soft-tissue mass in the right upper abdomen)
Solitary liver cyst (Hepatomegaly)
Solitary splenic cyst (Splenomegaly. Sometimes with cyst wall clcifications)

Splenic hematoma (Due to hematologic disorders or trauma)

Reference:18, 22, 26, 28, 30, 36, 44, 45, 53, 66, 71, 72, 111, 118, 120, 123, 130, 131
(See also Chapter 9, Table 1)

2. *Neonatal abdominal calcifications*
Abdominal wall:
 After subcutaneous emphysema
 Calcium salt injection
 Fat necrosis
 Generalized fibromatosis (Calcifications in the cutaneous lesions)
Peritoneal:
Meconium peritonitis (A sterile peritonitis secondary to perforation of the bowel proximal to an obstruction):
 Generalized
 Localized
Hydrometrocolpos (Accumulation of fluid within the obstructed uterus and/or vagina). May be associated with:
 Cloacal malformation (Single perineal orifice for the urinary bladder, vagina and rectum)
 Imperforate hymen
 Mayer-Rokitansky-Kuestner-Hauser syndrome (Uterus and vaginal agenesis with an intralabial mass)
 Persistent urogenital sinus
 Segmental vaginal atresia
Gastrointestinal:
Gastric bezoar (Concretions of foreign matter composed of accumulated ingested material in the gastrointestinal tract)
Infarcted bowel (Calcification of the involved segment)
Intestinal duplication cyst (A filling defect with calcification within the lumen of the cyst or in its wall):
 Duodenal
 Ileal
Intraluminal (Calcified meconium):
 Meconium in bowel
 Meconium in cloaca
 With anal atresia
 With multiple atresias
 Without distal obstruction
 Total aganglionosis

Intraluminal contrast agent:
  After amniography
  Transplacental maternal urography injection
Intramural bowel obstruction (Due to irreversible ischemia)
Hepatic:
Primary tumor:
  Hamartoma
  Hemangioendothelioma (Hepatomegaly with fine speckled calcifications)
  Hemangiomma (Peripheral-subcapsular in location, with calcifications - phlebolithes)
Metastatic tumor:
  Neuroblastoma (Hepatomegaly sometimes with tiny calcifications)
Neonata coxack-ivirus infection
Portal vein thrombosis (Hepato-splenomegaly with an enlatged azygos vein):
  Dehydration
  Perinatal omphalitis
  Post umbilical vein catheterization
Gallbladder:
Neonatal cholelithiasis
Total parenteral nutrition and furosemide treatment (Gallbladder stones)
Splenic:
Hematoma in hemophilia (Calcifications in the resolving hematoma)
Vascular:
Idiopathic arterial calcification
Inferior vena cava thrombosis
Portal vein thrombosis (Various etiologies)
Renal vein thrombosis (Various etiologies)
Retroperitoneum:
Adrenal:
  Hemorrhage (A suprarenal mass displacing the renal) May be associated with:....:
  Birth trauma
  Hemorrhagic disorders
  Hypoxia
  Infant of diabetic mother
  Septicemia (Various bacterial agents)
  Neuroblastoma (A suprarenal mass with stippled calcifications. Displacement of the kidney in an inferolaterally direction without distorsion of the collecting system)
  Wolman disease (Familial xanthomatosis. Enlarged adrenals with

Renal:
    Cortical necrosis
    Cystic disease:
        Cystic Wilms tumor
        Tuberous sclerosis
    Hydronephrosis (Various etiologies)
    Papillary necrosis
    Renal vein thrombosis (Various etiologies)
    Uriniferous perirenal pseudocyst (Urinoma. Varioue etiologies)
Teratoma
Scrotal:
Fat necrosis
Meconium peritonitis (Agregates of calcifications in the scrotum)
Teratoma (Dense calcifications with a radiolucent area)
Miscellaneous:
Amputated calcified ovary/ies (End result of torsion of an ovary. Calcification changes location with the change of the patient's position)
Fetus in fetus (Teratoma)
Ovarian dermoid (Tooth or bone equivalent calcification/s with a radiolucency [fat] in the pelvic region)

Reference: 18, 26, 36, 45, 66, 70, 75, 111, 118, 120, 123, 131
(See also Chapter 9, Table 23)

3. Bilateral renal mass/es in the newborn

Beckwith-Wiedemann syndrome (Organomegaly and accelerated bone age)
Bilateral hamartomas with tuberous sclerosis (Bilateral, multiple, tumors with calcifications)
Bilateral hydronephrosis (Dilatation of the collecting systems of the urinary tract):
    Bilateral obstructive ureterocele
    Bilateral ureteropelvic obstruction
    Bilateral ureterovesical obstruction
    Bilateral double collecting system
    Posterior urethral valves
Bilateral multicystic dysplastic kidney disease (Large kidneys with lobulated contures. No excretion on intravenous pyelogram)
Bilateral renal tumors (Varioue entities)
Bilateral renal vein thrombosis (Flank masses with hematuria)
Bilateral Wilms tumor:

Mesoblastic nephroma (Fetal renal hamartoma. A benign tumor. Bilateral large masses replacing the renal parenchyma)
Nephroblastomatosis (Arises from undifferentiated metanephric blastema as nephroblastomatosis. Bilateral multiple nodules)
Fanconi anemia
Glycogen storage disease (Mainly hepatomegaly. Moderate, bilateral renomegaly without distorting the collecting systems)
Hereditary tyrosinosis
Infant of diabetic mother
Leukemia and Lymphoma (Large kidneys with smooth borders)
Lymphangioma
Medullary sponge kidney (Dysplastic dilatation of the papillary and medullary portions of the collecting ducts. Medullary calcinosis)
Multicystic dysplastic kidney with a contralateral hydronephrotic kidney
Polycystic disease (Infantile type. Bilateral enlarged kidneys with prominent fetal lobulation)

Reference: 18, 22, 26, 30, 35, 44, 45, 66, 111, 118, 120, 123, 130, 131

4. *Unilateral renal mass/es in the newborn*
Abscess—Single or multiple
Compensatory hypertrophy
Ectopic kidney:
    Crossed ectopia (The distal ureter of the crossed ectopic kidney inserts into the trigon on the side of its normal origin)
    Pelvic kidney
    Renal fusion (Puncake renal appearance of both kidneys)
    Renal malrotation (The collecting system is positioned ventraly with partial extrarenal location)
Fancini anemia
Hydronephrosis (Dilatation of the unilateral collecting systemsof the urinary tract with or without renal functional impairment):
    Double collecting system
    Obstructing upper moiety of a duplex system
    Posterior urethral valves
    Ureterocele with a double collecting system
    Ureteropelvic obstruction
    Ureterovesical obstruction

Mesoblastic nephroma (Fetal renal hamartoma. A large non-calcified renal mass distorting the collecting system)
Multicystic dysplastic kidney (A unilateral abdominal mass with a lobulated contour)
Nephroblatoma (Multilocular cystic nephroma. A unilateral-uinifocal well cicumscribed mass with calcifications in the periphery of the mass)
Polycystic kidney (Various etiologies)
Renal vein thrombosis (Hematuria. Appearance of an enlarged kidney with a smooth border):
    Birth trauma
    Dehydration
    Diarrhea
    Enterocolitis
    Infant of diabetic mother
    Left adrenal hemorrhage
    Polycythemia
    Prematurity
    Sepsis
Teratoma (Various entities)
Trauma

Reference: 18, 26, 30, 36, 44, 45, 66, 95, 101, 111, 118, 120, 123, 131

5. "Lucencies" by the total-body opacification-effect during the early phase of an intravenous pyelogram
Kidney and urinary tract:
Abscess
Dilated bladder
Fetal renal hamartoma
Hydronephrosis
Hydroureter
Multicystic dysplastic kidney
Necrotic Wilms tumor
Pyonephrosis
Renal cyst
Renal vein thrombosis (Various etiologies)
Adrenal gland:
Hemorrhage
Neuroblastoma with necrosis

Genital:
Hydro-hemato-metro-colpos
Ovarian cyst
Gastrointestinal:
Duplication cyst
Gastric dilatation
L oculated ascites
Mesenteric arterial thrombosis with infarction
Omental or mesenteric cyst,
Pancreatic pseudocyst
Volvulus with infarction
Hepatobiliary:
Choledochal cyst
Focal liver necrosis
Hemangioma with low perfussion
Hydropic cholecystitis
Liver abscess
Liver cyst
Lymphangiomatous hamartoma of the liver
Spleen:
Cyst
Rupture

Reference: 26, 28, 36, 44, 66, 120, 123, 131

6. Delayed nephrogram in the newborn
Bilateral hydronephrosis
Congenital lues
Lower nephron nephrosis or tubular necrosis:
    After dehydration
    Infant of diabetic mother
Tamm-Horsfall proteinuria (Precipitation of abnormal proteins into the tubules lumen)

Reference: 18, 26, 36, 44, 66, 120, 123, 131

7. Hydronephrosis in the newborn
Megacystic magaureter syndrome
Neurogeneic urinary bladder:

Atonic type (Lower motor neuron lesion. Lesion below the conus medullaris)
Spastic type (Upper motoe neuron lesion. Lesion above the conus medullaris)
Posterior urethral valves (Congenital folds of mucous membrane located in the posterior urethra distal to the verumontanum. On voiding cystourethrogram -vesicoureteral reflux, and a trabeculated bladder)
Prolonged massive reflux
Prune belly syndrome (Eagle Barrett syndrome. Absent or hypoplastic abdominal wall musculature. Large urinary bladder with urethral obstruction. Non-obstructive megaureters, hydronephrosis and renal dysplasia accompanied by undescended testis)
Ureteropelvic junction obstruction (Pelvicaliectasis without ureter-ectasis. Funel shaped pelvis):

Aberrant vessel to lower renal pole (Compressing the junction)
Fibrous band crossing the junction
High ureteral insertion
Mucosal fold in the upper ureter
Pelvic calculus
Ureterovesical obstruction (A serpentine ureter with a secondary obstruction at the ureteropelvic junction)

Reference: 18, 26, 39, 36, 44, 45, 66, 75, 111, 118, 120, 123, 131
(See also this Chapter, Tables 48, 49)

8. *Perirenal urinoma in the newborn: uni- or bi-lateral*

Pelviureteric obstruction (Severe. Various etiologies)
Posterior urethral valves (Congenital folds of mucous membrane located in the posterior urethra distal to the verumontanum. Severe vesicoureteral reflux, trabeculated bladder and a large urinary bladder)
Vesicoureteric obstruction (Severe)

Reference: 18, 26, 36, 66, 111, 118, 120, 123, 131

9. *Urinary bladder outlet obstruction in the male newborn*

Anterior urethral valves
Circumcision inflammation, stricture or stenosis
Neurogenic bladder associated with lumbosacral meningocele: (Disturbed inervation of the detrusor muscle by the parasymphathetic nerves):

Atonic type (Lower motor neuron lesion)
Spastic type (Upper motoe neuron lesion)

Posterior urethral valves (Congenital folds of mucous membrane located in the posterior urethra distal to the verumontanum)
Prolapsing ectopic ureterocele (A cystic ectasia of the subepithelial segment of the intramural ureter at the urinary bladder wall. Usually, from an upper moiety of the double collecting sysytem which inserts medial to the lower moiety ureter below the level of the trigone)
Single system ureterocele
Urethral diverticula (Congenital anomaly or aquired-traumatic formation)
Urethral duplication and stenosis (Congenital anomaly)
Urethral polyps
Urethral stenosis (Congenital anomaly or acquired)

Reference: 8, 18, 22, 26, 30, 36, 44, 45, 66, 111, 118, 120, 123, 131, 148
(See also this Chapter, Table 59)

10. *Kidney border-loss on the plain radiogram*
Congenital absence of kidney
Ectopic kidney:
    Crossed ectopia (The distal ureter of the crossed ectopic kidney inserts into the trigon on the side of its normal origin)
    Pelvic kidney
    Renal fusion (Puncake renal appearance of both kidneys)
    Renal malrotation
Hemorrhage after trauma
Perinephric:
    Abscess (Extension of a renal abscess through the capsule. Loss of the psoas margin and obscuration of the renal contour)
    Hematoma
Post nephrectomy
Technical factors
Tumor displacement (By a neighboring space-occupying lesion)

Reference:18, 26, 36, 66, 68, 95, 120, 123, 131

11. *Depression of renal the margin/s*
Chronic pyelonephritis (Indentation over the clubbed calyces)
Fetal lobulation (Notching between the normal calyces)
Splenic impression (Flattening of the upper, outer margin, of the left kidney)

Reference: 18, 26, 45, 66, 111, 118, 120, 123, 126, 131

12. **Local bulge in the renal contour**
Angiomyolipoma (Associated with tuberous sclerosis)
Pseudotumor
Simple renal cyst
Subcapsular abscess
Subcapsular hematoma

Reference: 18, 26, 36, 45, 66, 111, 118, 120, 123, 130, 131
(See also this Chapter, Table 38)

13. **Abdominal mass in a child**
Appendicial abscess (Right lower abdominal mass)
Choledochal cyst (Right upper abdominal mass of soft-tissue at the lower liver margin)
Cysts (Various entities)
Hemangioma
Hepatoblastoma (Hepatomegaly with coarse calcifications)
Hydronephrosis (Dilatation of the collecting systems of the urinary system):
>   Double collecting system
>   Posterior urethral valves
>   Upper moiety of a duplex system
>   Ureterocele with a double collecting system
>   Ureteropelvic obstruction
>   Ureterovesical obstruction

Neuroblastoma (Abdomial mass with orbital ecchymosis. A suprarenal mass with stippled calcifications. Displacement of the kidney without distorsion of the collecting system. Retroperitoneal extension. Liver and bone metastasis)
Ovarian teratoma (Immature derivatives of all three germ cell layes A large solid mass in the pelvic cavity with calcifications
Teratoma in the sacral region
Wilms tumor (Nephroblastoma. A palpable mass with hematuria. Compresses renal tissue, distorts the renal calyces with renal pelvic penetration)

Reference: 18, 22, 26, 28, 45, 66, 111, 118, 120, 123, 130, 131
(See also Chapter 9, Table 7, Chapter 14, Table 5 and Chapter17, Table 1)

14. **High position of kidney**
Diaphragmatic hernia (Absence of closure of the pleuroperitoneal fold):
>   Bochdalek hernia (A posterolateral defect in the in the diaphragm)

(Eventration)

Mass displacing kidney upwards

Omphalocele (A midline defect over the entire ventral abdominal wall with herniation of the intra-peritoneal viscera into the base of the cord)

Thoracic kidney (High position of the posterior segment of the diaphragme with the adjacent kidney beneeth it)

Reference: 18, 26, 36, 44, 66, 120, 123, 131

15. *Low position of kidney*

Adrenal hemorrhage:
    Hemorrhagic disorders
    Septicemia
    Trauma
Ectopic kidney:
    Crossed ectopia (The distal ureter of the crossed ectopic kidney inserts into the trigon on the side of its normal origin)
    Pelvic kidney
    Renal fusion (Puncake renal appearance of both kidneys)
Hepatomegaly (Various etiologies)
Metastasis (Supra-renal metastasis/es)
Neuroblastoma, ganglioneuroma, pheochromocytoma or carcinoma
Ptotic kidney (Downward displced kidney in the up-right position due to laxity of the ligaments fixation of the kidney)
Retroperitoneal hematoma
Rhabdomyosarcoma in the retroperitoneum
Splenomegaly (Various etiologies)

Reference: 18, 26, 36, 44, 45, 66, 111, 118, 120, 123, 130, 131

16. *Displaced kidney*

Abscess, peprinephric (Extension of a renal abscess through the capsule)

Clear-cell carcinoma (An expansile mass which may cross the midline and contain calcifications)

Contralateral kidney invasion by tumor

Ectopic kidney:
    Crossed ectopia
    Pelvic kidney
    Renal fusion

Renal malrotation
Hematoma (Within the kidny parenchyma):
    Blood discrasia
    Trauma
Hepatomegaly (Various entities)
Hydatid cyst (A cyst with wall calcifications)
Lymphoma (Multiple nodular masses or a single bulky tumor which may infiltrate from the retroperitoneal region)
Metastasis
Neuroblastoma or gangglioneuroma (Supra- renal masses)
Ptotic kidney (Downward displced kidney in the up-right position)
Retroperitoneal hematoma
Rhabdomyosarcoma of the retroperitoneal origin
Splenomegaly (Varioue etiologgies)
Teratoma in the retroperitoneum (A soft tissue-mass with calcifications and lucent areas of fat-tissue)
Transplanted kidney (Implanted in the lower abdomen with removal of the own kidneys)
Vertebral tumor projecting into the retroperitoneum

_____

Reference: 18, 30, 36, 44, 45, 66, 111, 118, 120, 123, 131

17. *Bilateral enlarged kidneys*
Acute glomerulonephritis (Inflammatory disease of the renal parenchyma)
Acute nephrotic syndrome (Various etiologies)
Acute pyelonephritis (An acute upper urinary tract infection with bacteria causing parenchymal, caliceal and pelvic inflammation. A persistent dense nephrogram with delayed opacification of the collecting sysytem)
Acute renal failure:
    Cortical necrosis (Varioue etiologies)
    Infection
    Papillary necrosis (Varioue etiologies)
    Renal vein thrombosis (Various etiologies)
    Tubular necrosis (Various etiologies)
Angiomyolipoma (Bilateral. In tuberous sclerosis)
Beckwith-Wiedemann syndrome (Organomegaly and accelerated bone age)
Benign or malignant disorders:
    Bilateral fetal renal hamartomatosis
    Burkitt lymphoma
    Leukemia

Metastases

Nephroblastomatosis (Multiple neoplastic nodules which arise from undifferentiated metanephric blastema)

Wilms tumor (Bilateral)

Bilateral double collecting system without obstruction

Congenital megacalicosis (Caliceal dilatation caused by hypoplastic medullary pyramids. Prominent fetal lobulation with reduced parenchymal thickness. An increased number of calices)

Developmental disorders:

    Duplex kidneys:

        Complicated by obstructive ureteroceles

        Simple urterocele

    Horseshoe kidney

    Obstructive urophathy

    Polycystic disease:

        Adult type

        Infantile type

        Medullary sponge kidneys—cystic type or of dysplastic disorders

    Reflux—severe, with distal obstruction

Fanconi anemia

Gaucher disease (A cerebroside lipidosis)

Glycogen storage disease (von Gierke disease)

Hemolytic uremic syndrome (Bloody diarrhea, hemolytic anemia and Thrombocytopenia. Acute renal failure)

Infectious mononucleosis

Leukemic or lymphatic infiltrations (Large kidneys with smooth borders)

Mesoblastic nephroma (Fetal renal hamartoma. A large non-calcified renal mass distorting the collecting system)

Mucopolysaccharidosis (A lysosomal storage disorder. A multisystem involvement including bones and reno-hepato—splenomegaly)

Nephroblastomatosis (Arises from undifferentiated metanephric blastema as nephroblastomatosis. Bilateral multiple nodules)

Nephrosis (Various etiologies)

Nephrotic syndrome (Various etiologies)

Niemann-Pick disease (A sphingomyelin lipidosis)

Renal venous thrombosis (Hematuria, anuria and hypertension. Appearance of enlarged kidneys with a smooth border):

    Birth trauma

    Dehydration

    Diarrhea

Enterocolitis
Infant of diabetic mother
Left adrenal hemorrhage (In left renal vein thrombosis)
Polycythemia
Prematurity
Sepsis
Sarcoidosis (Enlarged kidneys with calcifications)
Sickle-cell anemia (Smooth large kidneys with a normal urogram. But, may be complicated with papillary necrosis or renal scaring)
Tuberous sclerosis (Multiple bilateral angiomyolipomata)
Visceromegaly (Various etiologies)

Reference: 18, 26, 30, 36, 44, 45, 66, 111, 118, 120, 123, 126, 131

18. *Unilateral enlarged kidney*

Acute pyelonephritis (An acute upper urinary tract infection with bacteria causing parenchymal, caliceal and pelvic inflammation)
Angiomyolipoma (In tuberous sclerosis)
Compensatory hypertrophy of the contralateral kidney (In loss of the ipsilateral renal parenchyma and loss of renal functions. Various etiologies)
Crossed fused ectopic kidney
Duplex kidney, simple or complicated
Hemihypertrophy with benign ipsilateral nephroomegaly
Horseshoe kidney (A congenital anomaly where the two kidneys are joined by their lower poles through a parenchymal or fibrous isthmus)
Hydatid cyst (A cyst with wall calcifications)
Hydronephrosis (Dilatation of the unilateral collecting system):
  Posterior urethral valves
  Single system ureterocele
  Upper moiety of a duplex system
  Ureterocele with a double collecting system
  Ureteropelvic obstruction (Primary or secondary)
  Ureterovesical obstruction
Intrarenal abscess including tuberculoma
Mesoblastic nephroma (Fetal renal hamartoma. A large non-calcified renal mass)
Metastasis
Multicystic dysplastic kidney, with or without obstruction
Multilocular cyst
Neuroblastoma with direct invasion of the ipsilateral kidney

Perirenal abscess (Extension of a renal abscess through the capsule)
Perirenal hematoma
Polycystic kidney
Pyonephrosis (Pus in the dilated collecting sysytem secondary to an infected hydronephrosis. Delayed excretion or no excretion during the intravenous pyelogram)
Renal cell carcinoma
Renal cyst (A solitary simple cyst)
Renal venous thrombosis (Hematuria. Enlarged kidney with a smooth border and a diminished nephrogram):
>   Dehydration
>   Diarrhea
>   Enteroco;itis
>   Left adrenal hemorrhage (After trauma)
>   Polycythemia
Sepsis
Sarcoidosis (Calcifications in the enlarged kidney)
Subcapsular hematoma
Transplanted kidney (Usually located in the lower abdomen):
>   Occlusion of the feeding renal artery at the anastomoosis
>   Rejection
>   Tubular necrosis
Trauma with nephric or perinephric hemorrhage:
>   Battered child syndrome
>   Contusion
>   Hematoma
Ureteropelvic junction obstruction (Pelvicaliectasis with a funel shaped pelvis):
>   Aberrant vessel to lower renal pole (Crossing and compressing the junction)
>   Fibrous band crossing the junction
>   High ureteral insertion
>   Mucosal fold in upper ureter
>   Pelvic calculus
>   Ureterovesical junction obstruction
>   Urinoma (A perirenal pseudocyst due to atear in a continous functioning collecting sysytem):
>   Bladder outlet obstruction (Of long duration)
>   Calculus obstruction in the collecting systen
>   Penetrating trauma
>   Ureteral obstruction with back pressure
Wilms tumor (Nephroblastoma. A palpable mass with hematuria. Compresses the renal tissue, distorts the renal calyces with renal pelvic penetration)

Xanthogranulomatous pyelonephritis (Global enlargement of the kidney with a focal mass. Extension of the inflammatory process into the vicinity of the involved kidnney)

Reference:18, 26, 36, 44, 45, 66, 68, 75, 90, 95, 101, 111, 118, 120, 123, 130, 131

19. *Bilateral small kidneys*

After papillary necrosis (A faint nephrographic effect. Waste parenchymal thickness with clubed-shaped calyces and intraluminal filling defects. Ringlike or papillary calcifications)

Ask-Upmark kidney (Glomerular focal hypoplasia. Small kidneys with decreased number of papillae and calyces)

Atrophy following obstruction or reflux (Vesicoureteral reflux and intrarenal reflux. Parenchymal thinning. Contour depression especially at the kidney poles. Scar formation opposite the clubbed calyces.)

Chronic glomerulonephritis (Wasted parenchyma, normal papillae and calyces)

Chronic pyelonephritis (Irregular kidney borders. Ffocal parenchymal thinning and contour depression especially at the kidney poles. Scar formation with adjacent clubbed calyces)

Congenital obstruction (At various levels with increased intrarenal urinary pressure)

Cortical necrosis (In the late phase of the disease. Smooth borders with calcifications):

    Burns

    Dehydration

    Hemolytic uremic syndrome

    Renal transplant rejection

    Scleroderma (See below)

    Sepsis

    Snake bite

    Transfusion reaction

Cystic dysplasia

Hypoplastic kidneys (Congenital anomaly)

Laurence-Moon-Biedl syndrome (Obesity with hypogonadism)

Le-Jeune syndroma (Asphyxiating thoracic dysplasia. Bone dysplasia)

Lupus erythematous (Renal failure with small or normal kidney size)

Medullary cystic disease (Nephronophthisis.Salt wasting, uremia and anemia. Smooth kidney conturs and a thin parenchyma)

Medullary necrosis (Various etiologies)

Obstructive uropathy (Dilatation of the collecting systems of the urinary tract)
Periarteritis nodosa
Post irradiation
Prune belly syndrome (Eagle Barrett syndrrome. Absent or hypoplastic abdominal wall musculature. Large urinary bladder with urethral obstruction. Non-obstructive megaureters, hydronephrosis and renal dysplasia, accompanied by undescended testis)
Reflux nephropathy (With or without infected urine. Vesicoureteral reflux and intrarenal reflux. Parenchymal thinning and contour depression especially at the kidney poles. Scar formation at the adjacent clubbed calyces. Dilated ureter secondary to the reflux)
Renal artery stenosis—bilateral (Fibromuscular hyperplasia)
Renal vein thrombosis (Nephrotic syndrome. Small contracted kidneys):
  Birth trauma
  Dehydration
  Diarrhea
  Enterocolitis
  Infant of diabetic mother
  Polycythemia
  Sepsis
  Trauma
Scleroderma (Progressive interstitial fibrosis with atrophy. Renal failure. Cortical necrosis)

Reference: 18, 26, 36, 44, 45, 66, 111, 118, 120, 123, 131

20. Unilateral small kidney

After irradiation
Ask-Upmark kidney (Glomerular focal hypoplasia. A small kidney with decreased number of papillae and calices. Hypertrophied contralateral kidney)
Atrophy following obstruction (A small kidney with focal parenchymal thinning and contour depression especially at the kidney poles)
Chronic pyelonephritis (Irregular kidney borders. Focal parenchymal thinning and contour depression especially at the kidney poles. Scar formation with adjacent clubbed calyces)
Dysplastic, Hypolastic kidney (Congenital anomaly)
Ischemia
Papillary necrosis (Smooth contours with a thin cortex. Club-shaped calyces. Displaced collecting system with intraluminal filling defect/s). May be associated with:
  Diabetes mellitus

Obstructive uropathy
Pyelonephritis
Renal vein thrombosis
Sickle cell disease
Obstructive uropathy (Dilatation of the collecting systems of the unilateral urinary tract. Various etiologies)
Partial nephrectomy
Post irradiation
Reflux nephropathy reflux (With or without infected urine, vesicoureteral reflux and intrarenal reflux. Focal parenchymal thinning and contour depression especially at the kidney poles. Scar formation with adjacent clubbed calyces)
Tuberculosis (Autonephrectomy. Unilateral contracted kidney with calcifications)
Vascular obstruction:
    Arterial (Fibromuscular hyperplasia)
    Embolus
    Occlusion
    Venous (Renal venous thrombosis)

Reference: 18, 26, 36, 44, 45, 66, 111, 118, 120, 123, 130, 131

21. *Absent nephrogram: Uni- or bi- lateral (Nonfunctioning of kidney)*
Absent kidney
    After nephrectomy
    Congenital—
        Uni- or bi-lateral agenesis
Acute cortical necrosis (Enlarged smooth kidney border/s with a faint or absent nephrogram):
    Burns
    Dehydration
    Hemolytic uremic syndrome (Bloody diarrhea, hemolytic anemia and Thrombocytopenia. Acute renal failure. Slightly increased size of kidneys with a faint or absent nephrogram)
    Renal transplant rejection (Renal artery thrombosis)
    Sepsis
    Snake bite
    Transfusion reaction
Multicystic dysplastic kidney (A large kidney with a lobulated contour)
Renal artery thrombosis

Renal vein thrombosis (Hematuria. Appearance of an enlarged kidney/s with a smooth border and a faint nephrogram):
Birth trauma
Dehydration
Diarrhea
Enterocolitis
Infant of diabetic mother
Left adrenal hemorrhage
Polycythemia
Prematurity
Sepsis
Total ureteral obstruction (Delayed apperence of a faint nephrogram)
Trauma with avulsion at the renal vascular pedicle (No nephrogram)
Tumor (If invading or obstructing the renal artery—no nephrogran or a very faint)

Reference: 18, 26, 36, 44, 66, 120, 123, 131
(See also this Chapter, Tables 24, 25)

22. *Weak nephrogram: uni- or bi- lateral*
Acute glomerulonephritis (Inflammatory disease of the renal parenchyma with decreased renal functions)
Acute pyelonephritis (An acute upper urinary tract infection. Delayed opacification of the collecting sysytem and dilatation of the ureters).
Chronic renal failure (Various etiologies)
Diabetes insipidus
Inadequate contrast medium injection
Increased diuresis
Mediteranien anemia (Small kidneys with a smooth conturs and a thin parenchyma. Poor opacification of the collecting sysytem with persistent medullary striations)
Nephrolithiasis
Overhydration
Polyuria
Unilateral hydroureter with hydronephrosis
Unilateral trauma
Uremia

Reference: 18, 26, 36, 44, 66, 68, 95, 101, 120, 123, 126, 131

23. Persistent nephrogram: uni- or bi- lateral
Acute renal failure
Acute tubular necrosis
Acute ureteral obstruction
Glomerulonephritis
Hydronephrosis
Hypotension
Low cardiac output
Medullary sponge kidney
Nephrosis
Papillary or medullary necrosis
Polycystic kidney (Infantile type)
Pyelonephritis (acute)
Renal vein thrombosis
Tamm-Horsfall proteinuria
Ureteric obstruction
Vascular insult to kidney

Reference: 18, 26, 36, 44, 66, 120, 123, 130, 131

24. Bilateral absence of kidney or no excretion on the urogram
Agenesis of kidneys
Bilateral nephrectomy
Bilateral pelvic kidneys
Bilateral renal vein thrombosis
Chronic nephrotic syndrome:
    Hemolytic uremic syndrrome
    Microcystic disease of kidneys
    Neil-patella syndrome (Osteo-onychodysostosis. Bone dysplasia))
Nonfunctioning kidneys with severe obstruction to urine flow (Various entities)
Pseudohermaphroditism
Septicemia

Reference: 18, 26, 36, 44, 45, 66, 111, 118, 120, 123, 130, 131
(See also this Chapter, Table 21)

25. Unilateral absence, or no nephrographic effect
Absent kidney:

Congenital unilateral kidney
Postoperative
Calculus obstruction
Ectopic kidney or crossed fused ectopia
High kidney position after repair of omphalocele
Multicystic dysplastic kidney
Obstructive uropathy
Pelvic kidney
Pyonephrosis
Renal artery thrombosis
Renal vein thrombosis:
    Dehydration
    Infant of diabetic mother
    Infection
    Trauma
Subcapsular hematoma or abscess
Thoracic kidney
Traumatic avulsion of kidney
Tumor (Expansion with destruction of the renal parenchyma)
Xanthogranulomatous pyelonephritis

Reference: 18, 26, 36, 44, 45, 66, 68, 95, 101, 111, 118, 120, 123, 131
(See also this Chapter, Table 21)

26. *The cortical rim nephrogram*
Partial renal artery occlusion (Various etiologies)
Renal vein thrombosis (Various entities)
Severe urinary tract obstruction with hydronephrosis
Tubular necrosis

Reference: 18, 26, 66, 120, 123

27. *Striated nephrogram*
Acute pyelonephritis (Of bacterial origin)
Infantile polycystic kidney disease
Medullary sponge kidney (Various entities)
Renal contusion
Renal vein thrombosis (Various entities)
Tamm-Horsfall proteinuria

Reference: 18, 26, 36, 66, 120, 123, 126, 131
(See also this Chapter, Table 46)

28. *Renal cystic disease*
Acquired renal cystic disease:
    Infectious cysts (Bacterial, parasits)
    Medullary necrosis
    Pyelogenic cyst
Cystic medullary disease:
    Medullary sponge kidney
    Nephronophthisis (Juvenile)
Cystic tumors:
    Cystic renal cell carcinoma
    Cystic Wilms tumor
Neurocutaneous dysplasia:
    Tuberous sclerosis
Polycystic renal disease:
    Adult
    Infantile
Renal dysplasia
    Multicystic dysplastic kidney
    Segmental or focal renal dysplasia
Simple renal cyst:
    Intrarenal
    Paravelvic

Reference: 18, 26, 45, 66, 89, 90, 111, 118, 120, 123, 131

29. *Medullary nephrocalcinosis*
Bartter syndrome (Tubular disorder with electrolytic loss and hyperaldosteronism)
Cushing syndrome
Diabetes mellitus
Furosemid therapy (Of long duration)
Hyperparathyroidism
Hypervitaminosis D
Idiopathic hypercalcemia
Immobilization of long duration
Lesch-Nyhan syndrome

Medullary sponge kidney
Milk-alkali syndrome
Milk of calcium in a pyelocaliceal diverticulum
Oxalosis
Renal papillary necrosis (Various etiologoes)
Renal tubular acidosis
Renal papillary necrosis (Various entities)
Sarcoidosis

Reference: 18, 26, 36, 45, 66, 111, 118, 120123, 131

30. *Medullary sponge kidney*
Calyceal diverticulum
Caroli disease
Ehlers-Danlos syndrome
Medullary nephrocalcinosis (Various entities)
Normal variant

Reference:18, 36, 44, 45, 66, 104, 111, 118, 120, 123

31. *Cortical necrosis*
Burns
Dehydration
Hemolytic uremic syndrome (Bloody diarrhea. Slightly increase in the size of the kidneys with a faint or absent nephrogram)
Renal transplant rejection (Renal artery thrombosis)
Sepsis
Snake bite
Transfusion reaction

Reference: 18, 26, 66, 111, 118, 120, 123, 131

32. *Syndromes with cortical cysts*
Conradi syndrome(Chondrodysplasia punctata)
Dandy-Walker syndrome (A congenital brain malfornmation)
Le-June syndrome (Asphyxiating thoracic dystrophy)
Meckel-Gruber syndrome
Oro-facial-digital syndrome
Trisomy 13

Tuberous sclerosis
Turner syndrome
Zellweger syndrome (Cerebrohepatorenal syndrome)

———————————

Reference: 26, 133

33. *Papillary necrosis*
Asphyxia neonatorum
Dehydration
Diabetes mellitus
Drugs
Hemorrhagic shock
Hyperbilirubinemia
Obstructive uropathy
Pyelonephritis
Renal venous thrombosis (Various etiologies)
Shock
Sickle-cell anemia

———————————

Reference: 18, 24, 26, 36, 44, 66, 111, 118, 120, 123, 126, 131

34. *Unilateral renal mass*
Abscess, including tuberculoma
Arteriovenous malformation (A unifocal mass with calcifications and a displaced collecting system)
Cysts:
    Hydatid (A cystic mass with wall calcifications)
    Multiple (Various etiologies)
    Parapelvic (A spherical mass attached to the pelvis of soft-tissue density. Focal displacement of the anatomical structures)
    Polycystic:
        Adult type
        Infantile type
    Solitary serous
Duplex kidney (Of the obstructed type)
Fetal lobulation
Hamartoma (Associated with tuberous sclerosis)
Hematoma:
    Blood dyscrasia

Trauma
Hydronephrosis (Various etiologies)
Invasion of the kidney by tumor from:
    Adrenal
    Retroperitoneum
Metastasis
Pseudotumor (Various etiologies)
Renal cell cacinoma
Subcapsular mass:
    Abscess
    Hematoma
Wilms tumor

Reference: 18, 26, 36, 44, 45, 90, 111, 118, 120, 123, 130, 131
(See also this Chapter, Table 4 and Chapter 17, Table 1)

35. Bilateral renal mass
Adult polycycstic disease
Angiomyolipoma
Leukemia
Lymphoma
Nephroblastomatosis
Renal cell carcinima
Wilms tumor

Reference: 18, 26, 44, 45, 66, 111, 118, 120, 123, 130, 131
(See also Chapter, Table 3)

36. Inflammatory renal mass
Abscess(small, large, single or multiple)
Bacterial endocarditis with emboli
Carbuncle (A focal mass displacing the collecting sysytem)
Hydatid cyst with secondary bacterial infection
Tuberculoma (A large irregular cavity with papillary necrosis)
Xanthogranulomatous pyelonephritis (A focal renal mass with an absent nephrogram, dilated calyces and a contracted pelvis)

Reference:18, 26, 36, 4, 45, 111, 118, 120, 123, 126, 131, 149a-b

37. **Upper pole renal mass**

Adrenal cyst (As a remnent of a resorbed hemorrhage)
Adrenal tumor, carcinoma
Neonatal adrenal abscess
Neonatal adrenal hemorrhage (The mass displacing the renal axis with peripheral calcificatiojns))
Neuroblastoma (Of the cystic type)
Upper moyete of a nonfunctioning duplex system
Upper pole cyst of kidney
Wilms tumor)Of the cystic type)

Reference: 18, 26, 36, 44, 45, 66, 111, 118, 120, 123, 131

38. **Psudotumor of kidney**

Abscess or tuberculoma (A large irregular cavity with papillary necrosis)
Compensatory hypertrophy
Cyst
Dromedary hump (A subcapsular bulge in the mid portion of the lateral border of the left kidney)
Enlarged column of Bertin (True pseudotumor. An anatomical variation. A lateral bulge of the renal cortex continuous with the cortex)
Extrarenal, extraparenchymal calyceal system (In cases of a longitudinal renal axis rotation)
Fetal lobulation (Persistent cortical lobation with a depression located between the renal calyces)
Hamartoma
Hillar lip (A supra- or infra- hillar bulge in the region of the medial part of the kidney)
Lateral indentation of the renal sinus
Nodular compensatory hypertrophy (An area of uneffected tissue in the presence of a focal renal scarring):
    Infarction
    Reflux nephropathy
    Surgery
    Trauma
Upper pole duplex kidney (Nonfunctioning)

Reference: 18, 26, 36, 44, 45, 66, 111, 118, 126, 123
(See also this chapter, Table 12)

39. *Calyceal abnormalities*
Calyectasis:
    Generalized—
        Congenital megacalyces
        Diabetes insipidus
        Obstructive and nonobstructive uropathy
    Localized—
        Chronic atrophic pyelonephritis
        Compound calyx
        Obdtructive calyectasis
        Papillary necrosis
        Pyelocalyceal diverticulum
Opacification of the collectig tubules—
    Medulary sponge kidney
    Pyelorenal backflow
Papillary cavity—
    Calyceal diverticulum
    Papillary necrosis
    Tuberculosis

Reference: 18, 26, 45, 104, 111, 118, 123, 126

40. *Narrowing of the calyceal infundibulum*
Edema of kidney:
    Acute glomerulonephritis (Inflammatory disease of the renal parenchyma with decreased renal functions)
    Acute nephrotic syndrome
    Acute renal vein thrombosis (Hematuria. Enlarged kidney with a smooth border and a faint nephrogram):
        Birth trauma
        Dehydration
        Diarrhea
        Enterocolitis
        Infant of diabetic mother
        Left adrenal hemorrhage
        Polycythemia
        Prematurity
        Sepsis
Kidney infiltration:

Glycogenosis (Glycogen strorage disease. Various etiologies)
Leukemia, Lymphoma (Diffuse infiltration throughout the renal parenchyma)
Metabolic storage disease (Various entities).
Local fibrosis (From a previous local inflammatory process)
Polycystic disease (Adult type. Compression by the enlarged cystic formations)
Renal fibromatosis (Congenital generalized fibromatosis. Multiple focal fibrous lesions compressing the calyceal infundibulum)
Tuberculosis

Reference: 18, 26, 36, 44, 66, 120, 123, 126, 131

41. *Narrowing of calyces or renal pelvis—Extrinsic causes*
Abscess
Arteriovenous fistula (Forming a conglomerate of vessels)
Hamartoma
Hematoma
Intrinsic renal mass
Polycystic kidney
Solitary cyst
Tuberculosis infection

Reference: 18, 26, 36, 44, 45, 66, 111, 118, 120, 123, 131

42. *Wide collecting system*
Congenital primary megaureter (A wide ureter with a normal tapered distal end)
Distended urinary bladder
Infection (Due to the bacterial toxins)
Long standing obstruction in the past (Despite the relive of the obstruction - the dilatation persists)
Megacalycosis (Underdevelopment of the papillae)
Megacystis-megaureter syndrome
Obstructive or nonobstructive uropathy:
    Acute obstruction
    Chronic obstruction
    Upper pole moiety obstruction of a duplicated system
Pelvi-ureteric diverticulosis
Prune-belly syndrome
Pyelocalyceal diverticulum
Vesicoureteral reflux

Reference: 18, 26, 40, 66, 104, 120, 123, 126, 131

43. *Filling defect in the collecting system*
Aberrant vessel
Blood clot
Calculus (Opaque or non-opaque)
Cystitis cystica
Fungus ball (Of Candida infection)
Gas bubbles:
    Gas forming bacteria
    Iatrogenic
Polyp
Pyelitis cystica
Sloughed papilla

Reference: 18, 26, 66, 104, 111, 118, 120, 123, 131
(See also this Chapter, Table 45)

44. *Intra-luminal mass in the collecting system*
Aberrant papilla (Papilla without a calyx protruding into a major infundibulm)
Air bubbles
Blood clot
Inflammatory debri:
    Schistomiasis
    Tuberculosis
    Xanthogranulomatous pyelonephritis
Nonopaque calculi
Prominent mucosal fold/s
Submucosal hemorrhage
Tissue slough:
    Fungus ball (Candidiasis)
    Inspisated debri
    Papillaty necrosis
Vascular notching

Reference: 18, 26, 45, 66, 111, 118, 120, 123, 131
(See also this Chapter, Table 45)

45. *Filling defect in the renal pelvis*
Aberrant papilla
Air bubbles:
  Abscess
  After retrograde pyelography
  Diabetes mellitus
  Voiding cystourethrogram
Blood clot
Calculus (Nonopaque, opaque)
Incomplete filling during intravenous pyelogram
Infundibular vascular impression
Malignant tumor (Primary, secondary)
Overlying intestinal gas
Papillary necrosis
Polyp
Pus
Pyelitis cystica
Renal hematoma
Renal neoplasm
Vascular anomalies:
  Aneurysm
  Arteriovenous malformation
  Collateral circulation
  Dilated splenic vein (From portal hypertension)

Reference: 18, 26, 36, 44, 45, 66, 68, 75, 95, 101, 111, 118, 120, 123, 130, 131
(See also this Chapter, Table 44)

46. *Striated renal pelvis*
After relif of an obstruction with hydronephrosis (Various etiologies)
Distensibility in repeated obstruction
Inflammatory process
Vesicoureteral reflux

Reference: 18, 26, 36, 44, 66, 123, 126
(See also this Chapter, Table 27)

47. *Upper urinary tract obstruction (Partial or complete)*
Kidney:
Calyceal obstruction:
  Calculus
  Congenital—
    Extrinsic—Vascular
    Intrinsic—Papillary necrosis
  Tuberculosis (Irregular cavity/s with necrosis and infundibular narrowing)
Tumor:
  Carcinoma
  Wilms tumor
Ureteropelvic junction obstruction:
  Associated with duplex kidney
  Associated with horseshoe kidney and malrotated kidney
  Intermittent
  Neonate
Ureter:
Adhesions
Blood clot (In the lumen)
Calculi
Congenital ureterovesical obstruction
Ectopic ureter (The ureter drains a single excretory system with an ectopic extravesical orifice)
Ectopic ureterocele (Obstruction of the upper moiety of a double excretory system)
Functional:
  Increased urine flow
  Prune-belly syndrome (Eagle Barrett syndrrome. Absent or hypoplastic abdominal wall musculature. Large urinary bladder with urethral bstruction. Non-obstructive megaureters, hydronephrosis and renal dysplasia, ccompanied by undescended testis)
  Reflux (Incompetence of the ureterovesical junction. Various etiologies)
Hydrometrocolpos (Accumulation of secretions within an obstructed uterus and/or vagaina)
Inflammatory disease:
Appendicitis (A soft tissue mass in the right lower abdomen)
Bilharziasis (Ureteral dilatation due to fibrotic narrowing of the affected section of the ureter)
Crohn disease (The inflammatory process extends from the intestine and is surrounding and obstructing the ureter)

Osteomyelitis (Originating in the pelvic bones and spreading towards the urinary tract
Pelvic inflammatory disease (Various entities)
Tuberculosis
Neoplasm:
Genitourinary neoplasm (Various entities)
Lymphoma (Masses and enlarged lymph glands in the retroperitoneum)
Neuroblastoma (Metastasis which spread in the retroperitoneum)
Physiologic:
Full bladder
Chronic constipation
Polyps
Retrocaval ureter (The ureter swings medially over the lumbar pedicles passing behind the inferior vena cava with a proximal hydroureteronephrosis)
Retroperitoneal fibrosis (Fibrous tissue compressing the ureter/s. Gradual tapering of the ureter/s with medial deviation)
Single system ureterocele (A congenital prolapse of the dilated distal ureter and its orifice into the urinary bladder lumen at the norma anatomic location of the trigone)
Stricture
Valve (Acquired or congenital mucosal folds within the ureteral lumen)

Reference: 18, 26, 45, 66, 75, 89, 90, 111, 118, 120, 123, 131, 148
(See also this Chapter, Table 48)

48. *Uni- or bi-lateral hydronephrotic kidney/s*
Associated with urinary tract infection
Bilateral double collecting system
Bladder outflow obstruction (Various etiologies)
Chronic granulomatous disease
Cystic disease of the kidney
Ectopic ureterocele (Obstruction of the upper moiety of a double excretory system)
Lower pole reflux (In a double collecting system)
Multicystic dysplastic kidney with a hydronephrotic contralateral kidney
Neurogenic urinary bladder (Varioue etiologies)
Ovarian cyst (Compressing the ureter)
Posterior urthral valves
Reflux without obstruction

Renal calculi (Various entities)
Retroperitoneal fibrosis (Fibrous tissue compressing the ureter/s. Gradual tapering of the ureter/s with medial deviation)
Retroperitoneal lymphoma
Retroperitoneal metastasis/es
Retroperitoneal sarcoma
Retroperitoneal treratoma
Severe cystitis (Various etiologies)
Ureteropelvic obstruction (Various etiologies)
Ureterovesical obstruction or severe reflux (Various etiologies)
Urethral obstruction:
    Diverticulum
    Embryonic sarcoma or urogenital sinus
    Stricture
Valves:
    Anterior urethral
    Posterior urethral
    Within the ureter
Wilms tumor (With ureteric compression)

Reference: 8, 18, 22, 26, 36, 44, 45, 66, 75, 111, 118, 120, 123, 126, 131, 149a-b
(See also this Chapter, Tables 7, 47)

49. Uretero-pelvic junction obstruction
Aberrant vessel to the lower renal pole
Calculus at the junction
Damage by a passing calculus
Extrinsic compression
Fibrous band
High ureteral insertion into the pelvis
Mucosal fold at the junction
Renal cyst
Secondary fibrosis (Post-infection)
Secondary obstruction (Due to a dilated–serpentine ureter)
Trauma:
    Direct damage
    Hemorrhage, locally
Tumor invasion
Xanthogranulomatous pyelonephritis

Reference: 18, 26, 36, 44, 45, 66, 68, 75, 95, 101, 111, 118, 120, 123, 130, 131

50. *Renal calculi in children (General overview)*
Immobilization stones:
Immobilized, bed-ridden patient
Infection stones:
Escherichia coli
Klebsiella
Proteus
Pseudomonas
Staphylococcus
Inflammatory bowel disease:
Crohan disease
Medication-induced stones:
Furosemide therapy
Steroids
Radiolucent stones:
Cystine
Uric acid
    Lesch-Nyhan syndrome (Self-mutilation. A dopamine metabolic defect)
    Leukemia
    Lymphoma
Xanthine
Urinary stasis stones:
Calyceal diverticula
Congenital megacalyces
Medullary sponge kidney
Posterior urethral valves
Primary megaureter
Ureterocele
Ureteropelvic junction obstruction
Various:
Cystic fibrosis

Reference: Modified from 75

51. *Calcification(s) in the kidney*
Abscess (Of pyogenic origin)

Bartter syndrome (Tubular disorder with electrolytic loss and hyperaldosteronism)
Calcified abscess or tuberculoma
Calcified cyst
Calcified hematoma
Calcium intake (Over-dossis)
Congenital arterio-venous malformation
Cushing syndrome
Diabetes insipidus
Diuretic drugs (Long duration of treatment)
Echinococcal cyst
Furosemide therapy in neonates
Idiopathic hypercalcemia and hypercalciuria
Immobilization (Bed-ridden patients)
Lesch-Nyhan syndrome (Self-mutilation. A dopamine metabolic defect)
Medullary sponge kidney (Various entities)
Milk-alkali syndrome
Milk-of-calcium (In pyelocaliceal divertiulum)
Nephrocalcinosis:
    Aminoaciduria
    Ctstyinuria
    Drugs—
        Heavy-metal ingestion
        Sulfonamide
    Hyperparathyroidism (A metabolic disorder)
    Hyperphosphatasia (A metabolic disorder)
    Hyperthyroidism (A hormonal and metabolic disorder)
    Hyperuricemia
    Hypervitaminosis D (Treatment with an over-dosis of vitamin D)
    Oxalosis
    Renal tuberculosis
    Sarcoidosis
    Total parenteral hyperalimentation
    Xanthogranulomatous pyelonephritis
Parenchymal necrosis:
    Cortical necrosis
    Papillary necrosis
    Tubular acidosis
    Tubular necrosis
    Venous thrombosis
Renal infarct

Subcapsular-perirenal hematoma
Tumor calcification:
  Clear-cell carcinoma
  Dermoid or teratoma
  (Neuroblastoma)
  Osteolytic bone metastasis
  Wilms tumor
Xanthogranulomatous pyelonephritis (A large obstructive calculus)

Reference: 18, 26, 36, 44, 45, 75, 104, 111, 118, 120, 123, 131

52. *Obstruction or stricture of the ureter*
Abscess
Blood clot
Calculus (Opaque or non-opaque calculus)
Chronic granulomatous disease
Extrinsic pressure on ureter:
  Appendiceal abscess
  Metastasis
  Non-malignant conditions—
    Cysts
    Hematoma
    Megacolon (Marked dilatation of the sigma compressing the ureteres and/or the urinary bladder)
  Primary tumor of the ureter
Inflammatory bowel disease (Such as Crohn disease where the inflammatory process extends from the intestine and is surrounding and obstructing the ureter)
Intrinsic polyp or tumor
Periureteral inflammatory process
Retroperitoneal fibrosis (Fibrous tissue enveloping the ureter/s. Mmedial deviation of the ureters and hydro-uretro-nephrosis)
Retroperitoneal hematoma (Various etiologies)
Schistosomiasis
Stricture:
  After instrumentation
  Inflammation
  Postirradiation
  Postoperative
Thickened bladder wall
Tumor invasion or pressure:

Lymphoma
Rhabdomyosarcoma
Seminoma (Metastasis/es)
Ureterocele (Ectopic, orthotopic, single system)
Ureterovesical stenosis

Reference: 18, 26, 27, 36, 44, 45, 66, 75, 111, 118, 120, 123, 131, 148, 149a-b

53. *Ureterovesical junction stenosis*
Anommalous or ectopic ureter insertion (Congenital anomaly)
Intrinsic stenosis
Invasion by inflammatory mass or tumor
Stone impacted at the junction (Opaque or non opaque calculus)
Ureterocele (Simple or ectopic)

Reference: 18, 26, 36, 44, 45, 66, 75, 111, 118, 120, 123, 131, 148

54. *Patulus distal urteric orifice*
Congenital anomalies:
Ectopic ureter (The ureter drains a single excretory system with an ectopic extravesical orifice)
Lower moiety of a duplex system
Megacystis-megaureter
Iatrogenic:
Post surgery—
Ureteral stump after nephrectomy
Post biopsy
Post ureteroscopy
Incomplete maturation of the uretero-vesical junction (in neonates)
Infectious diseases (Associated with vesicoureteral reflux. Various etiologies)
Malposition of the catheter during voiding cystourethrocystography
Non-obstructive megaureter
Prune belly sybdrome (Eagale-Barret syndrome. Absent or hypoplastic abdominal wall musculature. Distended ureters with marked ydronephrosis Undescended testes)
Neoplasm:
Primary
Secondary
Neurogenic dysfunction:

Neurogenic bladder (Various etiologies)

Reference: 22, 26, 36, 45, 66, 103, 111, 118, 120, 126, 123, 131, 148, 149a-b

55. *Megaureter: unilateral or bilateral*
Diabetes insipidus (Urinary excretion of great amounts due to reduced vaso-pressin production)
Diverticles of the urinary bladder
Ectopic ureterocele (Obstruction of the upper moiety of a double excretory system. The ureter is tortous and dilated)
Infection (Atonia of the ureter wall due to the bacterial toxins)
Megacystis megaureter syndrome (Very severe reflux)
Megaureter (Primary. Megaloureter)
Neurogenic bladder (The hypertonic type)
Neuromuscular deficit:
    Meningocele
    Meningomyelocele
    Sacral agenesis
    Sacral dysplasia
    Tumor of sacrum
No organic obstruction
Polyuria:
    Acute diuresis
    Diabetes insipidus (See above)
    Infection
Posterior urethral valves
Prune-belly syndrome (=Eagle-Barrett syndrome. Absent or hypoplastic abdominal wall musculature. Large bladder and urachal remnant. Marked distended ureters and hydronephrotic- dysplastic kidneys. Undescended testes)
Retrocaval ureter
Retroperitoneal fibrosis
Ureter remaining wide after reliving of an obstruction
Ureteral obstruction (Urterovesical obstruction)
Ureterocele (Of the obstructive-ectopic type)
Urethral obstruction:
    Blood clot
    Calculus
    Valves
Urinary bladder outflow obstruction (Various etiologies)

Urinary tract infection (Various etiologies)
Vesicoureteral reflux (Various etiologies)

Reference: 8, 22, 26, 36, 40, 44, 45, 66, 75, 111, 118, 120, 123, 126, 131

56. *Dilatation of the ureter at the level of the bony pelvis*
Bladder outflow obstruction (Various etiologies)
Congenital segmental dilatation (As in megaloureter = Primary megaureter)
Neurogenic bladder (The hypertonic type)
Prune-belly syndrome (Eagle-Barrett syndrome. Absent or hypoplastic abdominal wall musculature with a large bladder. Distended ureters and dysplastic kidneys. Undescended testes. In a certain group of the syndrome—urethral atresia or obstruction)
Reflux, as with:
   Cystitis cystica
   Inflammation
Schistosomiasis (A parasitic infestation. Due to inflammatory-fibrotic changes at the site of infection)

Reference: 18, 26, 36, 44, 66, 120, 123, 126, 131

57. *Ureteral notching*
Congenital septa
Diverticles
Inferior vena cava obstruction (Compression on the ureteric wall while crossing the inferior vena cava)
Kidney ischemia
Lymphangiectasis)Dilated lymphatics are imprinting the ureteric wall)
Omphalocele repair (Fibrotic bands traversing the ureter originating prom the posterior retroperitoneal wall)
Periarteritis nodosa
Renal artery stenosis
Renal vein thrombosis
Varicosities around the ureter
Vascular malformation

Reference: 26, 36, 40, 44, 66, 123

58. **Vesicoureteral reflux**
Bladder outflow obstruction (Various etiologies)
Congenital reflux (Primary reflux. Abnormal tunneling of the distal ureter through the bladder wall)
Cystitis (Various etiologies)
Duplication with a non-obstructive ureterocele
Ectopic anus with urogenital anomalies
Ectopic ureteral orifice (Various entities)
Infection (Of a bacterial origin)
Intrinsic anomaly at ureterio-vesical insertion (Such as diverticulum)
Neurogenic bladder(Various etiologies)
Paraureteric diverticulum (Hutch diverticulum)
Post-passing stone at the uretero-vesical junction
Prune-belly syndrome (Eagle-Barrett syndrome. Absent or hypoplastic abdominal wall musculature. Large bladder. Marked distended ureters)
Urethral obstruction (Various etiologies)

Reference: 8, 18, 22, 26, 36, 40, 44, 66, 75, 120, 123, 126, 131, 148

59. **Lower urinary tract obstruction (Partial or complete)**
Bladder::
Bladder neck obstruction (Circular muscular hypertrophy)
Blood clot after trauma or operation
Calculus:
    Foreign body serving as a nidus for a stone formation
    Renal calculi passing into the bladder
    Urinary stasis
Cystitis (Various entities)
Duplication (A congenital anomaly)
Extrophy (Congenital anomaly)
Foreign body (such as a catheter)
Neoplasm:
    Rhabdomyosarcoma (Originating from the prostata or vagina)
Neurogenic urinary bladdrer (Of the spastic type)
Neurofibroma
Saccules and diverticula (Various etiologies)
Trigonal cyst (Usually associated with cystitis)
Trigonal cystitis (As a part of aurinary bladder bacterial infection)

Trigonal diverticulum (Hutch diverticulum in the urinarry bladder wall near the ureterovesical insertion)

    Ectopic (The upper moiety ureter inserts inferior and medial to the lower moiety uretr, below the level of the trigone. In the male it inserts proximal to external ssphincter [No wetting], in the female- it may inserts also infra sphincteric [Wetting])

    Single system (Congenital prolapse of the dilated distal ureter and orifice into the urinary bladder at the usual location at the trigone. Seen with a single ureter. On the voiding urethrocystography, at the early stage of the bladder filling, the bulbus terminal ureter is demonstrated as a "cobra head" with a radiolucent halo around)

Posterior urethra:

Calculus

Cloacal anomaly

Ectopic prolapsing ureterocele (Obstructing the outflow tract)

Ectopic ureter (Ureter draining a single system with an ectopic extravesical orifice, or a urter draining an upper pole of a duplex system and exits below the urethral sphincter)

Muellerian duct anomaly:

    Cyst (A large cyst which extends cephald above the prostate and may obstruct the urethra if inflammed or infected)

    Mass

    Remnant (A cystic duct remnant of the para-mesonephric duct)

Polyp

Prune-belly syndrome (Eagle-Barrett syndrome. Absent or hypoplastic abdominal wall musculature. Large bladder and ureters. Undescended testes. In a certain group of the syndrome—urethral atresia or obstruction)

Rectourethral fistula (A congenital anomaly or an aquired fistula. Due to an inflammatory process or instrumentation)

Rhabdomyosarcoma of prostate (Penetrating the urethra or the trigonal area of the urinary bladder)

Stricture:

    Acquired—Instrumentation

                Post inflammation

Utriculus masculinous (Dilatation of the prostatic utricle. A cyst above the prostate gland with obstruction of the urethra)

Valve/s (Posterior urethral valves)

Anterior urethra:

Calculus

Cowper gland cyst

Diverticulum (In the anterior part of the urethra):
  Congenital
  Traumatic
Duplication (Congenital anomaly)
Foreign body in the urethra
Meatal stenosis (Aquired or congenital)
Megaurethra
Phimosis
Stricture:
  Congenital
  Inflammatory
  Traumatic
Valve/s (In the anterior part of the urethra. Consists of a mucosal fold)

Reference: 8, 18, 26, 45, 66, 75, 84, 89, 103, 111, 118, 120, 123, 131, 148
(See also this Chapter, Table 9, Tables 60, 70)

60. *Large urinary bladder appearance*

Bartter syndrome (A metabolic disorder with polyuria)
Bladder diverticula (True or pseudo-diverticulae of various etiologies)
Bladder outflow obstruction (Varioue etiologies)
Diabetes insipidus (Decreased vasopressin production with polyuria)
Megacystis megaureter syndrome
Megacystis—microcolon syndrome (Functional obstruction of the urinary bladder and colon)
Neurogenic bladder (Of the flaccid type)
Prune-belly syndrome (Eagle-Barrett syndrome. Absent or hypoplastic abdominal wall musculature with a large bladder. Distended ureters and hydro-nephrotic-dysplastic kidneys associated with undescended testes)
Psychogenic retention of urine
Reflux of severe primary type (Incompetence of the ureterovesical junction due to abnormal tunneling of the distal ureter through the bladder wall)
Rhabdomyosarcoma (Originating from the prostate gland or vagina, with an outflow obstruction of the urinary bladder)
Ureterocele (Of the ectopic-prolapsing type obstructing the outflow tract of the urinary bladder)
Urethral obstruction of any other cause

Reference: 18, 26, 36, 44, 45, 66, 111, 118, 120, 123, 126, 131
(See also this Chapter, Table 59)

61. *Small urinary bladder appearance*
After irradiation or chemotherapy
Bilateral renal agenesis (No urine production)
Bladder diversion
Bladder duplication (Congenital anomaly)
Cystitis, acute (Reduced urinary bladder capacity)
Cystitis cystica (Chronic infection. Reduced capacity because multiple small cystlike mucosal elevations)
Hemorrhagic cystitis
Intravesical cyst
Leukemic infiltration (Thick wall diminishig the pliability of the urinary blsdder)
Neurogenic bladder (Of the spastic type)
Pelvic hematoma (Compressing the bladder from the outside)
Repair after bladder extrophy
Schistosomiasis (Thick-walled fibrotic urinary bladder with high insertion of the ureters and reduced bladder)
Urinary diversion with isolation of the urinary bladder

Reference: 18, 26, 36, 44, 45, 66, 84, 111, 118, 120, 123, 131

62. *Neurogenic urinary bladder*
(Disturbance in the innervation of the detrusor muscles in the urinary bladder. The **atonic type**: Lower motor neuron lesion—lesion below the conus medullaris
The **spastic type**: Upper motor neuron lesion—abow the conus medullaris)
Aneurysmal bone cyst (An expansile lesion located in the lumbar spine)
Benign tumor involving the upper motor neuron
Cerebral palsy
Chordoma (A presacral osteolytic midline mass)
Diastematomyelia (Split cord. Sagital division of the spinal cord into two hemicords. In the region of the upper lumbar-lower thoracic spine)
Ependymoma (Tumor in the lower spinal cord)
Ewing sarcoma (Metastasis to the vertebra/e and spinal cord)
Infection of the spinal cord
Intraspinal lipoma (Associated with tethered cord)
Leukemia

Metastasis
Minor tauma to the cord in hemophilia
Myelomeningocele (In the lumbo-sacral region)
Neuroblastoma (Originating from the sympathetic chain which is extra- adrenal in location, and penetrating into the spinal canal through the intervertebral foramina)
Neurofibromatosis (A tumor of the nerve sheath)
Sacral agenesis, hypoplasia or dysgenesis (As a part of the caudal regression syndrome with hypoplasia of the distal spinal cord)
Sacral and/or coccygeal teratoma or dermoid cyst (May be associated with spinal dysraphism or sacral agenesis)
Spina bifida with meningocele or meningomyelocele (Of the lumbar region)
Spinal cord injury
Spinal cord tumor
Spinal epidural abscess
Trauma

Reference: 18, 26, 36, 44, 66, 68, 75, 95, 101, 120, 123, 131

63. *Urinary bladder wall thickening or a trabeculated bladder*
Cystitis (Various etiologies)
Neurogenic bladder (Various etiologies)
Partial voiding of the urinary bladder
Urinary bladder outlet obstruction (Various etiologies)

Reference: 18, 26, 45, 84, 111, 118, 120, 123, 126, 131

64. *Diverticle/s of the urinary bladder in children*
After reimplantation
Associated with ureterocele
Bladder outlet obstruction (Because of the increased pressure within the bladder there are formations of pseudodiverticulae. Herniation of the mucosa beetwin the trabeculations) is associated with:
     Posterior urethral valves
     Prolapsing ureterocele
     Rhabdomyosarcoma of the trigonal area
     Urethral stricture
Congenital diverticula (True diverticle/s. Contract on bladder voiding)
Cutis laxa (A disease of connective tissue with abnormal collagen synthesis)

Diamond-Blackfan syndrome
Ehlers-Danlos syndrome (A congenital disease of abnormal collagen formation)
Hutch diverticulum (Located in the paraureteral region):
  With reflux
  Without reflux
Kinky hair syndrome (Menkes syndromme)
Multiple diverticulae (Congenital or acquired)
Neurogenic dysfunction
Obstruction (Outflow tract obstruction with increased intravesical pressure)
Prune-belly syndrome (Eagle-Barrett syndrome. Absent or hypoplastic abdominal wall musculature. A large bladder and urachal remnant. Marked distended ureters and hydronephrotic- dysplastic kidneys)
Remnant of a rectovesical fistula
Site of a suprapubic tube
Urachal diverticulum
Ureteral stump (After nephrectomy)
Ureterocele remnant (After punctering of the ureterocele)
Williams syndrome (Idiopathic hypercalcemia. Elfinlike facies with cardio-vascular anomalies)

Reference: 18, 26, 36, 45, 66, 111, 118, 120, 123, 131

65. *Space-occupying lesion/s, filling defect/s or wall mass/es of the urinary bladder*
Blood clots
Calculus (Various etiologies)
Chronic granulomatous disease (Immunodeficiency disorder with granuloma formation in the urinary bladder wall)
Cystitis (Dysuria and hematuria):
  Abacterial cystitis
  Bullous cystitis
  Cystitis cystica (Multiple small round cyst-like mucosal elevations)
  Cytotoxic cystitis (A hemorrhagic cystitis after tumor theraphy)
  Edematous cystitis
  Emphysematous cystitis (A translucent ring of air bubbles in the bladder wall)
  Eosinophilic cystitis
  Hemorrhagic cystitis (Intraluminal blood clots)

Interstitial cystitis (Irregular mucosal pattern)
Malacoplakia
Embryonic sarcoma (Rhabdomyosarcoma. Penetrating from the prostata or vagaina forming the "sarcoma botryoides appearance") Foreign body Hemangioma (Protruding into the bladder lumen with phleboliths)
Hematoma (A soft-tissue mass with calcification protruding into the blader lumen)
Leukemic infiltration (Irregular wall protrusions into the lumen)
Metastasis
Neurofibroma
Papilloma
Polyps
Schistosomiasis (Multiple inflammatory pseudopolyps protruding from the bladder wall into the lumen secondary to granulomas - Bilharziumas)
Ureterocele (ectopic, simple)

Reference:18, 26, 45, 66, 68, 75, 84, 95, 101, 111, 118, 120, 123, 126, 130, 131, 148, 149a-b

66. *Calcifications in the urinary bladder*
After urinary bladder augmentation
Calculus:
  Foreign body in the bladder serving as the nidus to form a calculus
  Renal calculi passing into the bladder
  Urinary stasis in the bladder
Hemangioma (Congenital vascular malformation with phleboliths)
Hematoma (Calcified within the bladder)
Idiopathic hypercalcemia (Williams syndrome. Elfinlike facies with cardiovascular anomalies)
Immobilization
Insufficient water intake in hot regions
Neurogenic bladder (Stasis of urine)
Oxalosis (A metabolic disorder)
Schistosomiasis (Calcifications of the pseudopolyps and the eggs of the parasit)

Reference: 18, 26, 36, 44, 45, 66, 75, 111, 118, 120, 123, 131

67. *Filling defects in the (urinary) ileal-loop after diversion*
Adenocarcinoma (Developing from the ilial wall)

Calculus
Polyp (Developing from the ilial wall)
Prolapse of ureter
Vilous adenoma

Reference: 26, 44, 66, 75, 123

68. *Urinary bladder displacement*
From the front:
Hemangioma (A solitary compressible mass with phleboliths)
Metastasis
Pubic bone lesions (Tumors arising from the pubic and ischial bones)
From behind:
Abscess
Anterior meningocele (Arising from the lumbo-sacral region)
Chordoma (Bone tumor arising from the anterior aspect of the sacrum)
Distended colon (Feces)
Duplication of rectum (Congenital anomaly)
Ectopic anus with fistula and gut distension (Congenital anomaly)
Ectopic megaureter (Inserting below the external sphincter of the urethra with stenosing at its junction)
Foreign body in the vagina
Habitual constipation
Hemangioma (Soft-tissue mass with phleboliths)
Hematoma:
    Blood discrasia
    Hematoma
    Surgery
    Trauma
Hemato-metro-colpos or hydro-metro-colpos (Distension of accumulated fluid or secretion in the vagina and uterus)
Hirschsprung disease (Distension of the colon from above the narrow rectal segment)
Metastasis
Muellerian duct cyst (A large cyst which extends in the cranial direction above the prostate gland)
Neurofibromatosis
Neurogenic tumors (Arising from the nerve plexus located on the sacrum)

Pelvic neuroblastoma (Originating from the organ of Zuckerkandl and extendes caudaly behaind the urinary bladder)

Rhabdomyosarcoma (Originated from the striated muscular components of the posterior pelvic wall)

Sarcoma of the vagina or prostate gland (Extending towards the rectum)

Teratoma (A soft-tissue mass with a various degree and shape of calcifications)

Venous anomalies (A soft-tissue mass with phleboliths)

From the side:

Aneurysm, mycotic (From the iliac arteries)

Bladder diverticulum (Varioue etiologies)

Dilated veins

Direct extension from a pelvic bone tumor

Distended colon (Varioue etiologies)

Hematoma:
    Blood discrasia
    Hematoma
    Surgery
    Trauma

Inguinal hernia

Lymphadenopathy

Pelvic abscess (From pelvic inflammatory disese)

Sacral meningocele

Tumor of the innominate bone

From below:

Hematoma:
    Blood discrasia
    Hematoma
    Surgery
    Trauma

Pelvic floor abscess (From pelvic inflammatory disese or disemination from an intraperitoneal inflammatory-infected process)

Sarcoma of the prostate gland or vagina

Urine leak after trauma

Vascular anomalies

From above:

Ectopic kidney with tumor

Mesenteric cyst, large

Ovarian mass(An ovarian cyst)

Ureter (Grossly dilated)

Reference: 17, 18, 26, 36, 44, 45, 66, 68, 101, 111, 118, 120, 123, 131

69. *Mass in the Cul-de-sac*
(See also Chapter 19, Table 3)

70. *Urethral obstruction*
(The examination of choice is the micturition urogram)
Blood clot
Calculus
Diverticulum of urethra (anterior or posterior diverticulum)
Ectopic ureterocele (Prolapsing into the posterior urethra)
Embryonic sarcoma (Originating from the prostata or vagina and penetrating
into the posterior urethra)
Foreign body
Hydro-metropcolpos (The distended vagina compresses the urethra)
Meatal stricture or stenosis (Congenital or acquired)
Penile trauma
Phimosis
Posterior urethral valves
Post-traumatic stricture
Stenosis or atresia of urethra (Congenital or acquired)
Trauma to urethra
Urethral duplication (Congenital anomaly)
Urethritis
Valves:
   Anterior
   Posterior
Web (Congenital anomaly or a late result of an inflammatory process)

Reference: 8, 17, 18, 26, 36, 44, 66, 68, 75, 95, 101, 120, 123, 131
(See also this Chapter, Table 59)

71. *Causes of hematuria*
Acute glomerulonephritis
Acute renal vein thrombosis
Calculus disease
Coagulopathies
Cystitis hemorrhagica
Foreign body
Hemolytic uremic syndrome (Bloody diarrhea, congestive heart failure)
Idiopathic

Medullary cystic disease
Nephrocalcinosis:
    Cortical nephrocalcinosis
    Medullary nephrocalcinosis
Papillary necrosis
Polycystic disease (Adult type)
Polyps in the urinary tract
Renal cortical necrosis
Sarcoma invading bladder
Trauma
Urinary tract infection
Wilms tumor

Reference: 18, 26, 36, 44, 45, 66, 68, 75, 95, 101, 111, 118, 120, 126, 123, 131

72. *Renal vein thrombosis*
Cyanotic heart disease
Dehydration
Diarrhea
Hemoconcentration
Infant of diabetic mother
Invasion by Wilms tumor
Nephrotic syndrome
Sepsis
Shock state
Trauma

Reference: 18, 26, 36, 44, 45, 66, 111, 118, 120, 123, 130, 131

73. *Acute renal failure*
Congenital:
Bilateral renal agenesis, or dysplasia
Congenital nephritis
Congenital nephrotic syndrome
Infantile polycystic disease
Perinatal hypoxia
Postrenal:
Tumor of the bladder or retroperitoneum
Calculus obstruction

Prerenal:
Cardiac failure
Fluid and electrolyte depletion
Hemorrhage
Hepatorenal failure
Sepsis
Renal:
Arterial or venous obstruction
Burns
Cortical necrosis
Drug reaction
Glomerulonephritis (Acute stage)
Goodpasture syndrome (Pulmonar hemorrhage or pulmonary edema associated with acute renal failure)
Hemolytic uremic syndrome (Bloody diarrhea, congestive heart failure)
Hemo- or myo- globinuria
Papillary necrosis
Pyelonephritis
Radiographic contrast media
Schoenlein-Henoch purpura
Subacute bacrerial endocarditis
Trauma

Reference: 18, 26, 36, 45, 66, 111, 118, 123, 131

74. Chronic renal failure
Alport ysndrome (Progressive renal failure with proteinuria and hematuria)
Bilateral renal vein thrrombosis
Chronic glomerulonephritis
Chronic pyelonephritis
Hepato-renal syndrome
Hydronephrosis (Long standing obstruction or non-obstruction)
Infantile nephrotic syndrome
Medulary cystic disease
Multicystic dysplastic kidney
Polycystic kidney disease
Reflux nephropathy

Reference: 18, 26, 36, 45, 66, 111, 118, 120, 123,

75. **Polycythemia (Of renal origin)**
Obstructive uropathy
Polycystic kidney disease
Simple cyst
Vascular impairment
Wilms tumor

Reference: 26, 45, 66, 111, 118, 123

76. **Hypertension in childhood**
After irradiation of the kidney region
After renal operation
Arterio-venous fistula
Ask-Upmark kidney (Segmental renal hypoplasia)
Coarctation of the aorta (Abdominal or thoracic)
Dysmorphic kidney
Essential hypertension
Familial dysautonomia (Riely-Day syndrome)
Hemolytic uremic syndrome
Hydronephrosis
Neuroblastoma
Periarteritis nodosa
Pheochromocytoma
Polycystic renal disease
Renal artery stenosis
Renal parenchymal disease:
    Acute glomerulonephritis
    Anaphylactoid purpura
    Atrophic or chronic pyelonephritis
    Chronic glomerulonephritis
    Collagen vascular disease
    Cortical necrosis
    Medullary necrosis
    Nephrotic syndrome
    Scaring
    Urinary tract obstruction or obstructive uropathy
Renal vein thrombosis
Reno-vascular disease:
    Arterio-venous malformation
    Congenital stenosis by a fibrous band

Fibromuscular hyperplasia
Neurofibromatosis
Pheochromocytoma
Rubella syndrome
Takayasu syndrome (Pulseless disease)
Thrombosis:
 Renal artery
 Renal vein
Trauma:
 Avulsion of the renal vascular pedicle
 Occlusion of the renal vessels
Tuberous sclerosis
Vasculitis
Wilms tumor

Reference: 18, 26, 36, 44, 45, 66, 111, 118, 120, 123, 131

Chapter 16

The Adrenal Gland

(Nowadays the examination of choice is ultrasonography. The plain aabdominal film is complemantary to the sonographic examination)

1. *Adrenal gland mass*
Abscess
Cyst
Ganglioneuroma
Hemorrhage (After trauma, septicemia or other various etiologies)
Neuroblastoma:
    Cystic
    Solid
Pheochromocytoma
Tumor of cortex, carcinoma
Wolman disease (Lipidosis with adrenal calcifications)

───────────
Reference: 18, 26, 36, 45, 66, 68, 95, 101, 118, 120, 123, 131
(See also Chapter 15, Tables 1, 37)

2. *Bilateral large adrenal glands*
Hemorrage
Hyperplasia
Pheochromocytoma
Waterhouse-Friderichsen syndrome (A meningococcal septicemia)

───────────
Reference: 18, 26, 36, 44, 45, 66, 111, 118, 120, 123, 131

3. *Adrenal gland cortical diseases*
Adenoma

Adrenogenital syndrome
Cushing syndrome
Hyperplasia

Reference: 18, 26, 36, 44, 45, 66, 111, 118, 120, 123

4. Adrenal gland medullary disease
Ganglioneuroblastoma
Ganglioneuroma
Neuroblastoma
Pheochromocytoma

Reference: 18, 36, 44, 45, 66, 111, 118, 120, 123, 131

5. Adrenal gland calcifications
Addison disease (Chronic adrenal insufficiency)
Adenoma
Ganglineuroma
Hemorrhage–Post bleeding (Various etiologies)
Neuroblastoma
Pheochromocytoma
Sepsis
Tuberculosis
Tumor of the cortex
Waterhouse-Friderichsen syndrome (A meningococcal septicemia)
Wolman disease (Lipidosis with adrenal calcifications)

Reference: 18, 26, 36, 44, 45, 66, 68, 111, 118, 120, 123, 131

6. Polycythemia (Of adrenal gland origin)
Cushing disease
Pheochromocytoma

Reference: 26, 45, 66, 118, 123

Chapter 17

The Retroperitoneal Space

(Nowadays the examination of choice is abdominal ultrasonography. The plain aabdominal film is complemantory to the sonographic examination)

1. Retroperitoneal abdominal mass
Adrenal
Compensatory hypertrophy of kidney
Hematoma (Post-trauma)
Hydronephrosis
Lymphangioma
Lymphoma
Metastasis (Mainly from a testicular malignancy)
Multicystic kidney
Neuroblastoma
Renal venous thrombosis
Rhabdomyosarcoma
Solitary cyst
Teratoma
Ureteropelvic junction obstruction
Wilms' tumor

Reference: 18, 26, 36, 44, 45, 66, 68, 95, 101, 111, 118, 120, 123, 131
(See also Chapter 13, Table 1 and Chapter 16, Table 1)

2. Pneumoretroperitoneum
Disected mediastinal air
Gas abscess in the pancreas
Psoas muscle abscess
Traumatic rupture (Duodenal loop)

Urinary tract gas:
  Iatrogenic (Retrograde examination)
  Infection
  Trauma

_____

Reference: 18, 26, 66, 123

3. *Widening of the paraspinal soft tissues*
Abscess in the psoas muscle
Ganglineuroma
Lipomatosis
Lymphangioma
Lymphoma
Metastasis
Neuroblastoma
Sarcoma of various origin (Rhabdomyosarcoma of the psoas muscle)
Wilms tumor

_____

Reference: 18, 26, 32, 36, 45, 66, 111, 118, 120, 123, 131
(See also Chapter 2, Table 50 and Chapter 7, Table 19)

4. *Enlargement of the iliopsoas compartment*
Appendicitis
Coagulopathies (Bleeding into the compartment)
Complicated pancreatitis
Crohn disease (Extension of the inflammatory disease)
Discitis
Fluid colection:
  Pancreatic pseudocyst
  Urinoma
Hematoma (Post-trauma)
Lipomatosis
Lymphoma
Normal variation in the psoas muscle shape
Pelvic inflammatory disease
Renal infection
Retroperitoneal sarcoma
Spinal osteomyelitis

_____

Reference: 18, 26, 45, 66, 68, 74, 83, 95, 111, 118, 120, 123, 131

5. *Retroperitoneal calcifications*

Calcified hematoma (After trauma or surgery)
Cavernous hemangioma (Phleboliths of varius size and shape)
Hydatid cyst (Egg shall calcification/s)
Neuroblastoma (Fine granular calcifications)
Teratoma (Bone-like or teeth-like calcifications)
Tuberculous psoas abscess (Disorganized calcifications)
Wilms tumor (Amorphus calcifications of various sizes due to necrotic tumor tissue)

Reference: 18, 26, 36, 44, 45, 66, 111, 123, 131
(See also Chapter 13, Table 4)

Chapter 18

The Male Genital Organs

(Although ultrasonography is the examination of choice the conventional radiography is complemantery in those cases where the sonographic-wave can not analyze the pathologic process)

1. Ambiguous genitalia
Female pseudohermaphroditism (Masculinized extragenitalia but with a normal vagina, uterus and ovaries. Karyotype—46XX)
Male pseudohermaphroditism (Feminized ambiguous genitalia with undescended testes)
Mixed gonadal dysgenesis (Testes and gonadal streaks are identified and the uterus is usually present. Karyotype 46 XY)

Reference: 18, 26, 36, 45, 66, 111, 118, 120, 123

2. Acute scrotal disease
(Scrotal swelling and pain)
Acute epididymitis
Orchitis
Strangulated hernia
Testicular trauma
Torsion of testicular appendages
Torsion of testis

Reference:18, 26, 45, 111, 118, 123, 131

3. The scrotal mass
Calcifications (Various entities)
Cysts
Hematoma

Hydrocele
Inflamation
Scrotal hernia
Spermatocele
Tumor:
    Benign
    Malignant
Torsion
Varicocele

Reference: 18, 26, 36, 45, 66, 111, 118, 123, 131

4. *Scrotal wall thickening*
Complication of peritoneal dialysis
Complication of ventriculo-peritoneal shunt
Epididymo-orchitis
Henoch-Schoenlein purpura
Scrotal edema
Testicular torsion
Torsion of epididymal appendage
Torsion of testicular appendage
Trauma

Reference: 17, 18, 26, 36, 45, 66, 111, 118, 120, 123, 131

5. *Calcifications in the male genital tract*
Prostate
Seminal vesicles
Testicle/s
Vas deference

Reference:18, 45, 66, 111, 118, 123

6. *Calcifications within the scrotum*
Calcifications within the testis:
    Dermod
    Tumoral calcifications
Calcified hematoma
Meconium calcifications

Seminal vesicles
Vas deference

Reference: 18, 36, 45, 66, 111, 118, 120, 123, 131

Chapter 19

The Female Genital Organs

(Ultrasonography is the examination of choice for the female sexual organs. The conventional radiography may be complemantery analyzing the pathological process)

1. Hydro- hemato-metrocolpos
Blind horn of a bicornuate uterus (A congenital anomaly)
Cloacal malformation (A single perineal orifice for the urinary bladder, vagina and rectum)
Ectopic anus
Imperforate hymen
Mayer-Rokitansky-Kuester-Hauser syndrome (Agenesis of the uterus and vagina. Primary amenorrhea and an interlabial mass)
Peristent urogenital sinus (A single exit chamber for the urinary bladder and vagina. May be associated with ambiguous genitalia)
Sacral abnormalities
Transverse vaginal septum
Urinary anomalies with an ectopic ureter
Vaginal atresia or membrane

Reference: 18, 26, 36, 45, 66, 111, 118, 120, 123, 131

2. Adnexal mass
Tubo-ovarian abscess
Dermoid cyst (A congenital tumor containing mature tissues from all three germ cell layers with predominance of theectodermal components)
Ectopic pregnancy (Implantation outside the endometrial cavity)
Hydrosalpinx

Ovarian cyst
Teratoma of ovary (Immature derivatives of all three germ cell layers. A soft-tissue mass in the pelvis)

Reference: 18, 26, 36, 45, 63, 111, 118, 120, 123, 131
(See also Chapter 9, Table 72)

3. *Mass in Cul-de-sac*
Abdominal trauma (Ascitic fluid of various components)
Abscess (From a pelvic inflammatory disease)
Ectopic kidney
Ectopic ureter (Inserting into the urethra below the external sphincter with obstruction)
Fluid filled loops od small bowel
Hydro=hemato-metrocolpos (Distention of vagina and /or uterus by accumulated secretion)
Hydroureter
Intraperitoneal blood
Large normal uterus
Leiomyosarcoma
Lymphoma
Neurogenic bladder
Ovarian tumor
Pelvic inflammatory disease
Peritonitis
Pregnancy (Extrauterin pregnancy)
Rhabdomyosarcoma
Ruptured appendicial abscess
Ruptured bladder or rectum (From instrumentation or trauma)
Teratoma
Twisted ovary

Reference: 18, 26, 27, 36, 44, 45, 66, 68, 95, 111, 118, 120, 123, 131
(See also Chapter 15, Table 69)

4. *Polyhydramnios*
(Of the pregnant mother—suspected organ/s or systemic anomalies in the newborn)
Cardiac anomalies:
Arrhythmia
Ectopia cordis

Truncus arteriosus
Ventricular septal defect
Chest anomalies:
Chylothorax
Cystic adenomatoid malformation
Diaphragmatic hernia
Mediastinal teratoma
Pulmonary hypoplasia
Sequestration of lung
Tracheal atresia
Gastrointestinal anomalies:
Duodenal obstruction
Esophageal atresia
High intestinal atresia
Meconium peritonitis
Omphalocele
Genitourinary malformations:
Mesoblastic nephroma (Unilateral)
Multicystic dysplastic kidney (Unilateral)
Uretro-pelvic junction obstruction (Unilateral)
Neural tube defects:
Agenesis of corpus callosum
Anencephaly
Encephalocele
Holoprosencephaly
Hydranencephaly
Microcephaly
Myelomeningocele
Skeletal dysplasia:
Achondroplasia
Kyphoscoliosis
Platyspondyly
Thanatophoric dysplasia
Trisomy 13, 18, 21
Miscellaneous:
Amniotic band syndrome
Cleft lip aand/or cleft palate
Cystic hygroma
Teratoma

Reference: 18, 26, 66, 118, 120, 123, 131

5. *Oligohydramnios*

(Of the pregnant mother—suspected organ/s or systemic anomalies in the new-born)

Cloacal anomalies
Infantile polycystic kidney disease
Intrauterine growth retardation
Posterior urethral valves
Postmaturity
Premature rupture of membranes
Prune belly syndrome
Renal agenesis or dysgenesis
Urethral atresia

Reference: 18, 26, 66, 118, 120, 123, 131

Chapter 20

References

1. Adamsbaum C, Cohen PA, Carel JC (2000)
    Imaging strategies in endocrinopathies.
    Pediatric radiology. The state of the arte in 2000. Syllabus
    21:55-60 23rd Post-gradiate Course of the European Society of
    Pediatric radiolog.
    Springer Verlag, Milan

2. Alford BA, McIlhenny J (1999)
    An approach to asymmetric neonatal chest radiographh
    Radiol Clin North Am 37:1079-1092

3. Arenas-Jimenez JJ, Gomez-Fernandez-Montes J, Mas-Estelles E,
    Cortina-Orts H (1999)
    Large choledochocoele: difficulties in radiological diagnosis
    Pediatr Radiol 29:807-810

4. Aviv RI, Rodger E, Hall CM (2002)
    Craniosynostosis
    Clin Radiol 57:93-102

5. Babyn P (1999)
    Imaging follow-up of bone neoplasia.
    Highlights of Pediatric Radiology. Syllabus 17:57-63
    22nd Post-graduate Course of the European Society of Pediatric
    Radiology. Springer Verlag, Milan

6. Bagchi K, Mohaideen A, Thomson JD, Foley LC (2002)
    Hardware complications in scoliosis surgery.
    Pediatr Radiol 32:465-475

7. Bar-Ziv J, Koplewits BZ, Agid R (2001)
   Imaging of foreign body aspiration in the respiratory tract.
   International pediatric radiology. Post graduate course. Syllabus
   24:129-131
   4th International Pediatric Radiology Postgraduate Course.
   Springer Verlag, Milan

8. Bates DG, Coley BD (2001)
   Ultrasound diagnosis of the anterior urethral valve.
   Pediatr Radiol 31:634-636

9. Bernstein S, Weinstein M, Connolly B, Temple M (2001)
   Subcutaneous emphysema in a pediatric patient after radiologic
   placement of a percutaneous gastrostomy tube.
   Amer J Roent 177:693-694

10. Bhatt R, Rickett A (2000)
    Salmonella colitis: a mimic of Hirschprung disease.
    Pediatr Radiol 30:431

11. Blitman NM, Ali M (2002)
    Idiopathic giant esophageal ulcer in an HIV-positive child.
    Pediatr Radiol 32:907-909

12. Bloom DA, Buonomo C, Fishman SJ, Futura G, Nurko S (1999)
    Allergic colitis: a mimic of Hirschsprung disease.
    Pediatr radiol 29:37-41

13. Boechat MI, Winters WD, Hogg RJ, Fine RN, Watkins SL (2001)
    Avascular necrosis of the femoral head in children with chronic
    renal disease.
    Radiology 218:411-413

14. Brudnicki AR, Levin TL, Slim MS, Moser J, Amin N (2001)
    HIV-associated (non-thymic) intrathoracic lymphoepithelial cyst
    in a child.
    Pediatr Radiol 31:603-605

15. Buonomo C (1999)
    The radiology of necrotizing enterocolitis.
    Radiol Clin North Am 37:1187-1198

16.   Carty H (1999)
       Airway obstruction in children.
       Highlights of Pediatric Radiology. Syllabus 17:3-9
       22nd Post-graduate Course of the European Society of Pediatric
       Radiology. Springer Velag, Milan

17.   Carty H (2002)
       Sport injuries in children
       Postgraduate course. Syllabus 26:111-120
       25th Post-graduate Course of the European Society of Pediatric
       Radiology. Springer Verlag, Milan

18.   Carty H, Brunelle F, Shaw D, Kendall B (1994)
       Imaging Children.
       Churchill Livingstone, Edinburgh

19.   Cassar-Pullicino VN, Eisenstein SM (2002)
       Imaging in scoliosis: What, why and how.
       Clinc Radiol 57:543-562

20.   Chalumeau M, Foix-Phelias L, Zuani P, Gendrel D,
       Ducou-de-Pointe H (2002)
       Rib fractures after chest physiotherapy for bronchiolitis or
       pneumonia in Infants.
       Pediatr Radiol 32:644-647

21.   Clapuyt Ph, Saint-Martin Ch, Malghem J, Rombouts JJ (2000)
       Pediatric hip disorders: Imaging findings in adulthood.
       Pediatric radiology. The state of the arte in 2000. Syllabus 21:65-66
       23rd Post-gradiate Course of the European Society of Pediatric radiolog.
       Springer Verlag, Milan

22.   Claudon M, Ben-Sira L, Lebowitz RL (1999)
       Lower pole reflux in children: Uroradiologic appearences and pitfalls.
       Amer J Roent 172:795-801

23.   Connolly SA, Connolly LP, Jaramillo D (2001)
       Imaging of sport injuries in children and adolescents.
       Radiol Clin North Am 39:773-790

24. Crowley JJ, Sarnaik S (1999)
    Imaging of sickle cell disease
    Pediatr Radiol 29:646-661

25. Currarino G (2000)
    Double-layered manubrium sterni in young children with dias-
    trophic dysplasia.
    Pediatr Radiol 30:404-409

26. Daehnert W (1996)
    Radiology review manuel
    Williams and Wilkins, Baltimore

27. Daneman A (1999)
    Imaging of the postsurgical pediatric abdomen.
    Highlights of Pediatric Radiology. Syllabus 17:83-85
    22nd Post-graduate Course of the European Society of Pediatric
    Radiology. Springer Verlag, Milan

28. Daneman A, Traubici J (2002)
    An approach to imaging cystic lesions in the abdomen in pedi-
    atrics Postgraduate course. Syllabus 26:8-9
    25th Post-graduate Course of the European Society of Pediatric
    Radiology. Springer Verlag, Milan

29. Daneman A, Navarro O (2003)
    Intussusception. Part 1: A review of diagnostic approach.
    Pediatr radiol 33:79-83

30. De Kerviler E, Guermazi A, Zagdanski A-M, Gluckman E, Frija J (2000)
    The clinical and radiological features of Fanconi's anemia.
    Clin Radiol 55:340-345

31. Donnelly LF (1999)
    Maximizing the usefulmess of imaging children with communi-
    ty-acquired pneumonia: Review.
    Amer J Roent 172:505-512

32.   Donnelly LF, Frush DP, Zheng J-Y, Bisset III GS (2000)
       Differentiating normal from abnormal inferior thoracic paraver-
       tebral soft tissues on chest radiography in children.
       Amer J Roent 175:477-483

33.   Donnelly LF (2001)
       Chest wall abnormalities in children.
       International peduatric radiology. Post graduate course.
       Syllabus 24:95-100
       4th International Pediatric Radiology Postgraduate Course.
       Springer Verlag, Milan

34.   Donoghue V (2000)
       The newborn chest updated.
       Pediatric radiology. The state of the arte in 2000. Syllabus
       21:32-36
       23rd Post-gradiate Course of the European Society of Pediatric
       radiolog.
       Springer Verlag, Milan

35.   Doria AS, Huang C, Makitie O, Thorner P, Kooh SW, Sochett E,
       Daneman A (2002)
       Neonatal, severe primary hyperparathyroidism: a 7 year clinical
       and radiological follow-up of one patient.
       Pediatr Radiol 32:684-689

36.   Ebel KD, Blickman H, Willich E, Richter E (1999)
       Differential Diagnosis in Pediatric Radiology
       Thieme, Stuttgart

37.   Emery KG (2002)
       Lap belt iliac wing fracture: a predictor of bowel injury in children.
       Pediatr Radiol 32:892-895

38.   Fenton LZ, Buonomo C, Share JC, Chung T (2000)
       Small intestinal obstruction by remnants of the omphalomesen-
       teric duct: findings on contrast enema.
       Pediatr Radiol 30:165-167

39.   Fenton LZ, Buonomo C (2000)
        Benign pneumatosis in children
        Pediatr Radiol 30:786-793

40.   Geller E, Wolfson B, Rabinovitch H (2000)
        Multiple pelvoureteric diverticulosis in a 1-month-old infant with a
        del(10p) chromosomal abnormality presenting with UTI and VUR.
        Pediatr radiol 30:398-309

41.   Golan I, Baumert U, Held P, Feuerbach S, Muzig D (2002)
        Radiological findings and molecular genetic confirmation of
        cleidocranial dysplasia.
        Clin Radiol 57:525-529

42.   Goyal M, Swanson KF, Konez O, Patel D, Vyas PK (2000)
        Malignant pleural mesothelioma in a 13-year old girl.
        Pediatr radiol 30:776-778

43.   Grayev AM, Boal DKB, Wallach Dm, Segal LS (2001)
        Metaphyseal fractures mimicking abuse during treatment for
        clubfoot.
        Pediatr Radiol 31:559-563

44.   Grunebaum M (1986)
        Differential Diagnosis in Pediatric Radiology.
        Karger, Basel.

45.   Grunebaum M (2001)
        Ultrasonography of Newborns, Infants and Children.
        Diyonon Pub. Tel-Aviv. (In Hebrew)

46.   Gupta M, Koste Sc, Hopkins KP ((2002)
        Radiologic appearance of primary jaw lesions in children
        Pediatr Radiol 32:153-168

47.   Habert J, Haller JO (2000)
        Iatrogenic vertebral body compression fracture in a premature infant
        caused by extreme flexion during positioning for a lumbar puncture.
        Pediatr Radiol 30:410-411

48. Haje S, Harcke HT, Bowen JR (1999)
    Growth disturbance of the sternum and pectus deformities: imaging studies and clinical correlations.
    Pediatr Radiol 29:334-341

49. Hechter S, Huyer D, Manson D (2002)
    Sternal fractures as a manifestation of abusive in children.
    Pediatr Radiol 32:902-906

50. Hedlund GL, Navoy JF, Galliani CA, Johnson Jr WH (1999)
    Aggressive manifestations of inflammatory pulmonary pseudo-tumor in children.
    Pediatr Radiol 29:112-116

51. Hentel K, Brill PW, Winchester P (2002)
    Spontaneous hemopneumothorax
    Pediat Radiol 32:457-459

52. Herman TE, Coplen D, Skinner M (2000)
    Congenital short colon with imperforate anus (pouch colon). Report of a case.
    Pediatr Radiol 30:243-246

53. Hernanz-Schulman M (1999)
    Imaging of neonatal gastrointestinal obstruction.
    Radiol Clin North Am 37:1163-1186

54. Hubbard AM (2001)
    maging of pediatric hip disorders.
    Radiol Clin North Am 39:721-732

55. Jaramillo D (1999)
    Benign tumors of the Epi/metaphysis
    Malignant tumors of the Dia/metaphysis
    Highlights of Pediatric Radiology. Syllabus 17:68-71
    22nd Post-graduate Course of the European Society of Pediatric Radiology. Springer Verlag, Milan

56. Jaramillo D (1999)
    Malignant tumors of the Dia/metaphysis

Highlights of Pediatric Radiology. Syllabus 17:77-80
22nd Post-graduate Course of the European Society of Pediatric
Radiology. Springer Verlag, Milan

57.   Jaramillo D (2002)
       Imaging of infection and tumor in children
       Postgraduate course. Syllabus 26:47-49
       25th Post-graduate Course of the European Society of Pediatric
       Radiology. Springer Verlag, Milan

58.   John SD (1999)
       Trends in pediatric emergency imaging.
       Radiol Clin North Am 37:995-1934

59.   Joshi A, Derdon WE, Brudnicki A, LeQuesne G, Ruzal-Shapiro
       C, Hayes C (2002)
       Gastric thumbprinting: diffuse gastric wall mucosal and submucos-
       al thickening in infants with ductal-dependent cyanotic congenital
       heart disease maintained on long-term prostaglandin therapy.
       Pediatr Radiol 32:405-408

60.   Jurriaans E, Singh NP, Finlay K, Friedman L (2001)
       Imaging chronic recurrent multifocal osteomyelitis.
       Radiol Clin North Am 39:305327

61.   Kalifa G (2001)
       Recent data on osteoporosis and disorders of calcium and
       phosphorus metabolism in children.
       International Peduatric Radiology. Post graduate course.
       Syllabus 24:87- 91
       4th International Pediatric Radiology Postgraduate Course. Springer
       Verlag, Milan

62.   Kamata S, Sawai T, Nose K, Hasagawa T, Nakajima K, Soh H,
       Okada A (2000)
       Extralobar pulmonary sequestration with venous drainage to
       the portal vein: a case report
       Pediatr Radiol 30:492-494

63. Karmazin B, Steinberg R, Ziv N, Zer M, I Horev G (2002)
    Colonic stricture secondary to torsion of an ovarian cyst.
    Pediatr Radiol 32:25-27

64. Katz M, Konen E (1999)
    Imaging of pediatric diseases of the tracheobronchial tree.
    Highlights of Pediatric Radiology. Syllabus 17:18-22
    22nd Post-graduate Course of the European Society of Pediatric
    Radiology. Springer Verlag, Milan

65. Kawano S, Tanaka H, Daimon Y, Niizuma T, Terada K, Kataoka N,
    Iwamura Y, Aoyama K (2001)
    Gastric pneumatosis associated with duodenal stenosis and
    malrotation.
    Pediatr Radiol 31: 656-658

66. Kirks DR, Griscom NT (1997)
    Practical Pediatric Imaging: Diagnostic Radiology of Infants and
    Children.
    3rd ed. Lippincott-Raven, Philadelphia

67. Kjellin IB, Boechat MI, Vinuela F, Westra SJ, Duckwiler Gr (2000)
    Pulmonary emboli following therapeutic embolization of
    cefebral arteriovenous malformations in children.
    Pediatr Radiol, 30:279-283

68. Kleinmen PK (2002)
    Imaging in child abuse: An update
    Postgraduate course. Syllabus 26:105-110
    25th Post-graduate Course of the European Society of Pediatric
    Radiology. Springer Verlag, Milan

69. Kogutt Ms, Lovretich JO (1999)
    Periosteal reaction of the long bones associated with extracor-
    poral membrane oxigenation: cause and effect.
    Pediatr Radiol 29:797-798 (Lettr to the Editor)

70. Konen O, Rathaus V, Bauer S, Dolfin T, Shapiro M (2000)
    Progressive liver calcifications in neonatal coxsack-ivirus infection.
    Pediatr Radiol 30:343-345

71.   Konen O, Rathaus V, Dlugy E, Freud E, Kessler A, Shapiro M, Horev G (2002)
      Childhood abdominal cystic lymphangioma.
      Pediat Radiol 32:88-94

72.   Koplewitz BZ, Daneman A (1999)
      The lateral view: a useful adjunct in the diagnosis of malrotation.
      Pediatr Radiol 29:144-145 (Letter to the editor)

73.   Koplewitz BZ, Ramos C, Manson DE, Babyn PS, Ein SH (2000)
      Traumatic diaphragmatic injuries in infants and children: imaging findings.
      Pediat Radiol 30:471-479

74.   Kothaxi NA, Pelchovitz DJ, Meyer JS (2001)
      Imaging of muskuloskeletal infections
      Radiol Clin North Am 39:653-671

75.   Kraus SJ, Lebowitz RL, Royal SA (1999)
      Renal calculi in children: Imaging features that lead to diagnoses: a pictorial essay.
      Pediatr Radiol 29:624-630

76.   Kurugoglu S, Mihmanli I, Celkan T, Akai H, Aksoy H, Korman U (2002)
      Radiological features in pediatric primary gastric MALT lymphoma and association with *Helicobacter pylori*.
      Pediatr Radiol 32:82-87

77.   Kwon DS, Spevak MR, Fletcher K, Kleinman PK (2002)
      Physiologic subperiosteal newbone formation: Prevalance, distribution, and thickness in neonates and infants.
      Amer J Roentgenol

78.   Lee MA, Marven S, Roberts JP, Sprigg A (2000)
      Neonatal duodenal stenosis and reflux into the biliary tree.
      Pediatr Radiol 30:433

79.   Liu ACY, Argent ID (2002)
      Necrobacillosis—A resurgence
      Clin Radiol 57:332-338

80.   Luedtke LM, Flynn JM, Ganley TJ, Hosalkar HS, PillSG, Dormans JP (2001)
       The orthopedist's perspective: bone tumors, scoliosis and trauma.
       Radiol Clin North Am 39:803-821

81.   Macedo F, McHuge, Goldblatt D (1999)
       Pricardial effusions in two boys with chronic granulomatous disease.
       Pediatr Radiol 29:820-822

82.   Mahboubi S, Glaser DL, Shore EM, Kaplan FS (2001)
       Fibrodysplasia ossificans progressiva
       Pediatr Radiol 31:307-314

83.   Mahboubi S, Morris MC (2001)
       Imaging of spinal infections in children
       Radiol Clin North Am 39:215-222

84.   McCarville MB, Hoffer FA, Gingrich JR, Jankins III JJ (2000)
       Imaging findings of hemorrhagic cystitis in pediatric oncologic patients.
       Pediatr radiol 30:131-138

85.   McHugh K (2001)
       Pulmonary tumors in childhood.
       International Pediatric Radiology. Post graduate course. Syllabus 24:151-153
       4th International Pediatric Radiology Postgraduate Course. Springer Verlag, Milan

86.   Mengozzi E, Sartoni-Galloni S, Giovannini G, Bronzetti C (2001)
       Mycotic aneurysm of the thoracic aorta presenting as pneumonia.
       Pediatr Radiol 31:488-490

87.   Miller SL, Hoffer FA (2001)
       Malignant and benign bone tumors (2001)
       Radiol Clin North Am 39:673-699

88.   Morrison SC, Laya B (2001)
       Colo-colic intussusception in an infant with pneumatosis.
       Pediatr Radiol 31:494-496

89. Murphy RC, Berdon WE, Ruzal-Shapiro C, Hall EJ, Kornecki A, Daneman A, Brunelle F, Campbell JB (1999)
Malignencies in pediatric patients with ataxia telangiectasia.
Pediatr Radiol 29:225-230

90. Narla LD, Hingsbergen EA, Jones JE (1999)
Adult diseases in children
Pediatr Radiol 29:244-254

91. Nazaroglu H, Mete A, Bukte Y, Simsek M (2002)
Agenesis of the right lung presenting as a pulmonary infection.
Clin Radiol 57:529-530

92. Newman B (1999)
"Face Lifting" of the newborn chest - Surfactant and extracorporal membrane oxygenation.
Highlights of Pediatric Radiology. Sylabbus 17:3-9
22nd Post-graduate Course of the European Society of Pediatric Radiology. Springer-Verlag, Milan

93. Newman B(1999)
Imaging of medical disease of the newborn lung
Radiol Clin North Am 37:1049-1065

94. Newman B, Kuhn JP, Kramer SS, Carcillo Ja (2001)
Congenital surfactant protein B deficiency—emphasis on imaging.
Pediatr Radiol 31:327-331

95. Nimkin K, Kleinman PK (2001)
Imaging of child abuse.
Radiol Clin North Am 39:843-864

96. Odita JC (2001)
The sifnificance of recurrent lung opacities in neonates on surfactant treatment for respiratory distress syndrome.
Pediatr Radiol 31:87-91

97. O'Malley M, Roche C (2001)
Cervical spine injury.

International Peduatric Radiology. Post graduate course. Syllabus 24:190-200
4th International Pediatric Radiology Postgraduate Course. Springer Verklag, Milan

98.   Oudjhane K, Azouz EM (2001)
       Imaging of osteomyelitis in children
       Radiol Clin North Am 39:251-266

99.   Owens C (2002)
       The radiology of difuse interstitial pulmonary diseases in children.
       Postgraduate course. Syllabus 26:133-142
       25th Post-graduate Course of the European Society of Pediatric Radiology. Springer Verlag, Milan

100.   Pursner M, Haller JO, Berdon WE (2000)
        Imaging features of Mycobacterium avium-intracellulare complex (MAC) in children with AIDS.
        Pediatr Radiol 30:426-429

101.   Rao P, Carty H (1999)
        Non-accidental injury: Review of the radiology.
        Clin Radiol 54:11-24

102.   Rathause V, Grunebaum M, Ziv N, et al. (1992)
        The bubble sign in the gasless abdomen of the newborn.
        Pediatr Radiol 22:106-108

103.   Rathaus V, Konen O, Shapiro M, Grunebaum M (2001)
        Malposition of catheters during voiding cystourethrography.
        Eur Radiol (2001) 11:651-654

104.   Rathhaus V, Konen O, Werner M, Shapiro-Finberg M, Grunebaum M, Zissin R (2001)
        Pyelocalyceal diverticulum: the imaging spectrum with emphasis on the ultrasound features.
        Brith J Radiol 74:595-601

105.   Remes VM, Helenius IJ, Marttinen EJ (2001)
       Manubrium sterni in patients with diastrophic dysplasia - radio-
       logical analysis of 50 patients.
       Pediatr Radiol 31:555-558

106.   Remes VM, Marttininen EJ, Poussa MS, Helenius IJ, Peltonen
       JI (2002)
       Cervical spine in patients with diastrophic dysplasia—radi-
       ographic findings in 122 patients.
       Pediat Radiol 32:621-628

107.   Ringertz HU, Lidegran m (1999)
       Mediastinal and hilar neoplasia in children.
       Highlights of Pediatric Radiology. Syllabus 17:23-26
       22nd Post-graduate Course of the European Society of
       Pediatric Radiology. Springer Verlag, Milan

108.   Roche C, Carty H (2001)
       Spinal trauma in children.
       Pediat Radiol 31: 677-700

109.   Rosendahl K (1999)
       Imaging of arthritis in children.
       Highlights of Pediatric Radiology. Syllabus 17:64-67
       22nd Post-graduate Course of the European Society of Pediatric
       Radiology. Springer Verlag, Milan

110.   Royal SA (2000)
       Pediatric laryngeal granular cell tumor.
       Pediatr Radiol 30:869-870

111.   Rumack CM, Wilson SR, Charboneau JW (1991)
       Diagnostic ultrasound, Vol 2, Pediatric ultrasonography.
       Mosby-Year book, St. Louis.

112.   Sakurai M, Donnelly LF, Klosterman LA, Strife JL (2000)
       Congenital diaphragmatic hernia in neonates: Variations in
       umbilical catheter and enteric tube position.
       Radiology 216:112-116

113. Sanderson E, Newman V, Haigh, Baker A, Sidhu PS (2002)
     Vertebral anomalies in children with Alagille syndrome: an
     analysis of 50 consecutive patients.
     Pediat Radiol 32:114-119

114. Schmit P, Prieur A-M, Brunelle F (1999)
     Juvenile rheumatoid arthritis and lympoedema: lymphangio-
     graphic aspects.
     Pediatr Radiol 29:364-366

115. Schulman H, Tsodikow V, Einhorn M, Levy Y, Shorer Z, Hertzanu
     Y (2001)
     Congenital insensitivity to pain with anhidrosis (CIPA): the spec-
     trum of radiological findings.
     Pediatr Radiol 31: 701-705

116. Schwartz DS, Reyes-Mugica M, Keller MS (1999)
     Imaging of surgical diseases of the newborn chest: Intrapleural
     mass lesions.
     Radiol Clin North Am 37:1087-1078

117. Shewchuk Jr, Reed MH (2002)
     Pediatric postprimary pulmonary tuberculosis.
     Pediatr Radiol 32:648-651

118. Siegel JM (Editor), (2001)
     Pediatric sonography.
     Lippincott-Raven, Philadelphia

119. Silengo M, Gianino P, Longo P, Battistoni G, Defilippi C (2000)
     Dandy-Walker complex in a child with Jeunes asphyxiating tho-
     racic dystrophy.
     Pediatr Radiol 30:430

120. Silverman FN, Kuhn JP (1999)
     Caffey's Pediatric X-ray Diagnosis: An Integrated Immaging Approach.
     9th Ed. Mosby, Chicago

121.   Slama M, Andre C, Huon C, Antoun H, Adamsbaum C (1999)
       Radiological analysis of hyaline membrane disease after
       exogenous surfactant treatment.
       Pediatr Radiol 29:56-60

122.   Spadola L, Anoshiravani M, Sayegh Y, Jequier S, Hanquinet S (2002)
       Generalized infantile myofibromatosis with intracranial involve-
       ment: imaging findings in a newborn.
       Pediatr Radiol 32:872-874

123.   Starshak RJ, Wells RG, Dty JR, Gregg DC (1992)
       Diagnostic Imaging of Infants and Children
       (Genitourinary system; Gastrointestinal system; Liver; Pancreas
       and Spleen).
       Aspen Pub. Inc, Gaithersburg (Vol. II)

124.   States LJ (2001)
       Imaging of metabolic bone disease and marrow disorders in children.
       Radiol Clin North Am 39:749-790

125.   Stay GS, Yousefzadeh (2000)
       Scapular duplication.
       Pediatr Radiol 30:412-414

126.   Stokland E (2002)
       Imaging in urinary tract infections: An update
       Postgraduate course. Syllabus 26:67-69
       25th Post-graduate Course of the European Society of Pediatric
       Radiology. Springer Verlag, Milan

127.   Strife JI, Sze RW (1999)
       Radiographic evaluation of neonate with congenital heart disease.
       Radiol Clin North Am 37:1093-1107

128.   Sty JR, Wells RG, Starshak RJ, Gregg DC (1992)
       Diagnostic Imaging of Infants and Children
       (Cranium and Brain; Spine; Extracranial Head and Neck).
       Aspen Pub. Inc, Gaithersburg. (Vol. I)

129. Sty JR, Wells RG, Starshak RJ, Gregg DC (1992)
      Diagnostic Imaging of Infants and Children
      (Cardiovascular system; Chest; Musculoskeletal system).
      Aspen Pub. Inc, Gaithersburg,. (Vol. III)

130. Swischuk LE, John SD (1995)
      Differential Diagnosis in Pediatric Radiology.
      2ed Ed. Lippincott, Williams & Wilkins, Baltimore

131. Swischuk LE (1997)
      Imaging of the Newborn, Infant, and Young Child.
      4th ed., Lippincott, Williams & Wilkins, Baltimore

132. Swischuk LE, John SD, Tschoepe EJ (1999)
      Upper tibial hyperextension fractures in infants: another occult
      toddler's fracture.
      Pediatr Radiol 29:6-9

133. Taybi H, Lachman RS (1996)
      Radiology of syndromes, metabolic disorders and skeletal dysplasia.
      4th ed. Mosby, St Louis

134. Torre M, Martucciello G, Jasonni V (2001)
      Sacral development in anorectal malformations and in normal
      population.
      Pediatr Radiol 31 858-862

135. Tortori-Donati P, Rossi A (2001)
      Brain tumors in children.
      International peduatric radiology. Post graduate course. Syllabus
      24:28-41
      4th International Pediatric Radiology Postgraduate Course.
      Springer Verlag, Milan

136. Tsai S-L, Crain EF, Silver EJ, Goldman HS (2002)
      What can we learn from chest radiographs in hypoxemic asthmatics.
      Pediatr Radiol 32:498-504

137. Turra S, Giante C, Pavanini G, Bardi C (2000)
     Spinal involvement in Pyle's disease.
     Pediatr Radiol 30:25-27

138. Umit Sarrici S, Yurdakok M, Unal S (2001)
     Acute gastric dilatation complicating the use of mydriatics in a
     preterm newborn.
     Pediatr Radiol 31:581-583

139. Varan A, Kutluk T, Demirkazik FB, Akyiiz C, Buyukpamukcu M (2000)
     Hypertrophic osteoarthropathy in a child with nasopharyngeal
     carcinoma.
     Pediatr Radiol 30:570-572

140. Vasquez-Mendez E, Piqueras J (2000)
     Neuroimaging of pediatric systemic diseases.
     International Peduatric Radiology. Post graduate course.
     Syllabus 24:22-27
     4th International Pediatric Radiology Postgraduate Course.
     Springer Verlag, Milan

141. Vazquez JL, Buonomo C, Nurko S (1999)
     Barrett's esophagus in a teenager with a ringed esophagus.
     Pediatr Radiol 29:641 (Letter to the Editor)

142. Vrdoljak J, Irha E (2000)
     Synovial osteochondromatosis of the sternoclavicular joint.
     Pediatr Radiol 30:181-183

143. Wihlborg CEM, Babyn PS, Schneider R (1999)
     The association between Turner's syndrome and juvenile rheuma-
     toid arthritis.
     Pediatr Radiol 29:676-681

144. Wihlborg C, Babyn P, Ranson M, Laxer R (2001)
     Radiologic mimics of juvenile rheumatoid arthritis.
     Pediatr radiol 31:315-326

145.   Williams HJ, Wake MJC, John PR (2002)
        Intraosseous haemangioma of the mandible: a case report.
        Pediatr Radiol 32:605-608

146.   Wootton-Gorges SL, Albano EA, Riggs JM, Ihrke H, Rumack CM,
        Strain JD (2000)
        Chest radiography versus chest CT in the evaluation for pul-
        monary metastases in patients with Wilms' tumor: a retrospec-
        tive review.
        Pediatr Radiol 30:533-539

147.   Wootton-Gorges SL, Eckel GM, Poulus ND, Milstein JM (2002)
        Duplication of the cervical esophagus: a case report and review
        of the litarture.
        Pediatr Radiol 32:533-535

148.   Zerin JM, Baker DR, Casale JA (2000)
        Single-system ureteroceles in infants and children: imaging fea-
        tures.
        Pediatr Radiol 30:139-146

149   a. Zi Yin E, Frush DP, Donnelly LF, Buckley Rh (2001)
        Primary immunodeficiency disorders in pediatric patients:
        Clinical features and imaging findings.
        Amer J Roent 176:1541-1552

        b. Manson DE, Sikka S, Reid B, Roifman C (2000)
        Primary immunodeficiencies: a pictorial immunology primer for
        radiologists.
        Pediatr Radiolo 30:501-510

Chapter 21

Index of the Various Iimaging Signs

(Abbreviations: **Chapter** = C ; **Table** = T)

Carpal aangle C1-T139
Clavicle C1-T110
Ileo-cecal valve C9-T71
Phalanges C1-T143
Radioulnar, proximal C1-T133
Ribs, segmentation C1-T119
Scapula C1-T116
Swallowing C9-T2, T28
Teeth growth C4-T33
Ulna C1-T137
Vertebrae C2-T3
Vocal cords C6-T37
Absence of
    Clavicle, lateral end C1-T111
    Diaphragmatic movements C7-T27
    Digits C1-T145
    Kidney
        Bilateraal C15-T24
        Unilateral C15-T25
    Lamina dura C4-T34
    Lyphoid tissue in nasopharynx C4-T50
    Main pulmonary artery segment C8-T44
    Nephrogram C15-T21, T25
    Patella C1-T170
    Ribs C1-T117
    Teeth C4-T31
    Thymus gland C7-T7
    Vertebral pedicle C2-T27
Acetabulum/ar
    Angle
        Large C1-T156
        Small C1-T155
    Protrusion C1-T160
    Triradiate C1-T157
Adenopathy
    Hilar, with anterior mediastinal fullness C7-T15
Adrenal gland
    Calcifications C16-T5
    Cortical disease C16-T3
    Large C16-T2

Vertebrae C2-T2
Bell-shaped thorax C7-T30
Benign defects, metadiaphyseal C1-T44
Benign pneumatosis C9-T96, C14-T9
Biconcave vertebra C2-T24
Bilateral
    Adenopathy
        Hilar, lung C6-T55
        Mediastinal C7-T15
    Central pulmonary opacification C6-T66
    Cyst, multiple, lung C6-T94
    Diaphragm, position
        High C7-T23
        Low C7-T25
    Hilar enlargement C6-T54
    Homogenous opacification of lung C6-T10
    Hydronephrosis C15-T48
    Hyperinflation C6-T13, T57
    Hypoinflation C6-T59
    Interstitial fibrosis, lung C6-T85
    Kidney
        Absence C15-T24
        Hydronephrosis C15-T7, T48
        Large C15-T17
        Small C15-T19
    Lung opacification C6-T102
    Lung opacification not confined to a lobe or segment C6-T68
    Maxillary sinus hypoplasia C4-T37
    Megaureter C15-T55
    Periosteal reaction, symmentric C1-T67
    Renal mass, newborn C15-T1
    Under aeration of lung C6-T59
    Widening of mediastinum C7-T10
Biliary tract, gas in C11-T3
Birth trauma
    Bone C1-T14
    Calvarium C3-T55
Block vertebrae C2-T6
Blured margins, epiphysis C1-T23
Body asymmetry C1-T185

Bone
    Absent sternum C1-T105
    Age
        Advanced C1-T70
            At birth C1-T11
            Later in life C1-T71
        Disharmonic C1-T74
        Retardation C1-T72
            At birth C1-T10
            Localized C1-T73
            Post-natal period C1-72
    Battered child C1-T91
    Bowing of long bones
        Isolated C1-T56
        Tibia C1-T171
    Bubbly or cystic lesion C1-T87
    Clavicle (See C1-T110-T115)
    Cortex
        Cyst like defects C1-T86
        Spliting C1-T53
    Decreased density C1-T77
    Defect, cortex C1-T54
    Diaphyseal
        Lesion C1-T47
        Tumor C1-T94
    Dysharmonic bone age C1-T74
    Dyaplasia
        Cyst-like defects C1-T86
        Fracture C1-T9
        Hyperostosis C1-T8
        Lethal C1-T1
        Osteosclerosis C1-T8
        Periosteal thickening C1-T60
        Potentially lethal C1-T2
        Viable C1-T4
    Epiphyseal
        Lesion C1-T25
        Tumor C1-T94
    Erosion/s of inner cortical margin C1-T52
    Exostosis, multiple or single C1-T101-T103

Expansile bone tumor C1-T96
Fracture
    Newborn C1-T14
    Pathologic C1-T92
    Scapula C1-T116
    Skull C1-T56
    Sternum C1-T105
Fussion
    Carpal bones C1-T140
    Sternum bones C1-T105
Growth
    Generalized increase of…C1-T75
    Isolated increase C1-T18, T76
    Localized retardation or arrest T1-T73
Humeral notch, proximal C1-T132
Increased density
    Generalized C1-T35
    Localized C1-T81
Infarct/s
    Diaphyseal C1-T57
    Meta-diaphyseal C1-T45
Length
    Increased C1-T75
    Isolated C1-T76
Long
    Overtubulation C1-T50
    Undertubulation C1-T49
Malformation, thorax C1-T104, C6-T27
Metacarpus, metatarsus, short C1-T141, T142
Metaphyseal lesion without marginal sclerosis C1-T41
Moth-eaten destructive lesion/s C1-T99
Multiple lesions in a single bone C1-T84
Osteoblastic metastasis C1-T98
Osteolytic, destructive lesions C1-T96, T99
Osteoporosis, osteopenia C1-T77
Osteosclerotic lesions, multiple C1-T82
Pathologic fracture C1-T92
Pelvis, ossification, abnormal C1-T154
Polyostotic lesions C1-T90
Primary bone tumor C1-T94-T96

Synostosis C3-T11
Thick
    Base C3-T21
    Bone C3-19
Thinning of skull bones C3-T24
Trigonocephaly C3-T12
Ventriculo-peritoneal shunt C3-T17
Wide sutures C3-T7, T8, T18
Wormian bones, increased number C3-T9
Craniolacunia C3-T25
Craniosynostosis C3-T11
Cul-de-sac C15-T69, C19-T3
Cupping metaphysis C1-T39
Cyanosis
    Decreased pulmonary arterial vasculature C8-T16
        Right aortic arch C8-T22
    Increased pulmonary arterial vasculature C8-T12, T15, T19
    Increased pulmonary venous vasculature C8-T17
    Newborns (see Newborns) C8-T1
    Respiratory distress C8-T2
Cyst
    Fluid levels in lung C6-T93, T94
    Intra-abdominal C9-T100
    Intrathoracic C6-T95
    Jaw C4-T22
    Lung, solitary C6-T93
    Mandible C4-T21
    Pulmonary, multiple C6-T91, T92
        With, without air-fluid level C6-T93
    Thorax C6-T95
Cyst-like
    Defects, bone C1-T86
    Structures in lung, parenchymal
        Childhood C6-T90
        Newborn C6-T18
Cystic
    Kidney disease C15-T28
    Lesions, bone C1-T86, T87

D
Decreased density
  Bone
    Osteoporosis, osteopenia C1-T77
Decreased interpediculate distance C2-T30
Defecation problems, newborn C9-T17
Defect
  Anterior abdominal wall, newborn C9-T6
  Bone, orbit C4-T10
  Cecum, filling defects C9-T73
  Duodenal bulb C9-T57
  Epiphysis C1-T25
  Filling, small bowel C9-T66
  Metaphysis, without marginal sclerosis C1-T41
Defective
  Skull ossification C3-T23
  Teeth growth C4-T32
Deformation
  Madelung C1-T138
  Terminal ileum C9-T67
  Vertebral, step C2-T7
Delay closure, cranial sutures C3-T8
Delayed nephrogram, newborn C15-T6
Dense
  Cranial bones C3-T18
  Orbital bones C4-T9
  Rib/s C1-T129
Density
  Increased
    Abdominal cavity C9-101
    Bone C1-T79, T81
    Epiphysis C1-T26
    Metaphysis C1-T35
    Vertebra
    Body C2-T20
    Pedicle C2-T28
  Inner upper wall of chest
    Newborn C6-T26
  Lung (See also Parenchyma)
    Nodule

Pseudodiverticulum, intramural C9-T38
Reflux, gastro-esophageal C9-T32
Stricture C9-T35
Swallowing, abnormal C9-T2, T28
Tracheo-esophageal communication C6-T41, C9-T40
Ulcer C9-T33
Varices C9-39
Wide C9-T36
Eye (See also Orbit)
    Orbit(al) cavity, shallow C4-T1
        Bone defect C4-T10
        Calcification C4-T5
        Dense bone C4-T9
        Exophthalmos
        Bilateral C4-T6
        Unilateral C4-T7
        Hypertelorism C4-T13
        Hypotelorism C4-T12
        Large C4-T4
        Mass C4-T8
        Optic foramen, large C4-T11
        Shape C4-T3
        Small C4-T1
Excavatum, pectus C1-T107, C7-T32
Excursion, disorder, diaphragm C7-T22
Exostosis
    Multiple C1-T101, T103
    Single C1-T101, T102
Expending medullary lesion, thin cortex, diaphysis C1-T96
Extracardiac causes for congestive heart failure C8-T11
Extrathoracic disease with pleural effusion C6-T112
Extraluminal rectosigmoid obstruction C9-T86
Extrinsic compression of esophagus C7-T9, C9-T41

F
Failure, congestive heart
    Extracardiac causes C8-T11
    Slightly enlarged heart C8-T61
Failure, renal
    Acute C15-73

Upper air-way obstruction C6-T28
Infarction of
    Bone
        Diaphyseal C1-T57
        Metadiaphyseal C1-T45
    Lung C6-T84
Infection, urinary tract
Infiltration of
    Liver, fatty, radiolucent C10-T5
    Lungs
        Patchy, asymmetric, alveolar C6-T17
        Pneumonia C6-T62
            Alveolar C6-T3, T63
            Reticular C6-T73
        Reticulo-nodular, newborn C6-T6
Inflammatory renal mass C15-T36
Infratentorial
    Calcification/s C3-T51
    Space occupying lesion C3-T53
Inner wall, chest density C6-T26
Interpediculate distance
    Decreased C2-T30
    Increased C2-T29
Interstitial (Lung)
    Emphysema, newborn C6-T12
    Fibrosis C6-T85
    Granulo-nodulo-alveolar pattern C6-T72
    Markings C6-T73
    Non-homogeneous opacification C6-T74
    Peribronchiolar C6-T56
    Pneumonitis, disseminated C6-T75
    Reticular pattern C6-T73
Intervertebral disc
    Calcifications C2-T46
    Narrowing C2-T45
    Widening C2-T44
Intestinal
    Gas, reduced C9-97
    Loops, increased distance between C9-98

Right lower abdomen with abnormal gas pattern C9-T72
Scrotal C18-T3
Thoracic wall soft-tissue, with or without rib involvement C7-T33
Upper pole of kidney C15-T37
Urinary bladder
    Filling defect C15-T65
    Wall C15-T65
Vertebral arch/body C2-T32
Mastoid
    Air-cells, opacification C4-T16
    Destructive lesions C4-T17
Maxillary sinus
    Hypoplasia, bilateral C4-T37
    Mass C4-T45
    Opacification C4-T40
    Sinusitis, chronic C4-T41
        Unilateral with nasal drainage C4-T42
Meconium plug syndrome C9-T19
Medial notch, humerus, proximal C1-T132
Mediastinum
    Adenopathy C6-T55, C7-T15
    Bi- or uni- lateral C6-T52, T54, T55
    Air in mediastinal shadow C7-T2
    Anterior mass C7-T13, T15
    Calcification/s C7-T28
    Differential diagnosis of soft-tissue band C7-T14
    Displacement C7-T3, T4
    Hilar adenopathy C7-T15
    Immunodeficiency disorders C7-T8
    Inferior posterior, paravertebral soft-tissue widening C7-T19
    Intrathoracic ectopia of abdominal organs C7-T20
    Middle, mass C7-T16
    Narrow C7-T6
    Mass
        Anterior C7-T13
        Hilar adenopathy C7-T15
        Between trachea and esophagus C7-T9
        Lower posterior thoracic mass C7-T18
        Middle C7-T16
    Pneumomediastinum C7-T1

Cyanosis
　Heart disease C8-T1
　Decreased pulmonary arterial vasculature C8-T13
　Increased pulmonary arterial vasculature C8-T12
　Respiratory distress C8-T2
Cyst-like structures in lung parenchyma C6-T18
Defectaion problems C9-T17
Disused colon C9-T22
Double bubble sign C9-T15
Fecal-gas pattern C9-T18
Fetal fluid retention C6-T4
Fracture, rib/s C1-T14, T15
Functional disorder of colon C9-T21
Gas in portal vein C9-T26, C10-T2
Gasless abdomen C9-T13
Gastric obstruction C9-T16
Hepatomegaly C10-T1, T4
Hollow viscus prforation C9-T24
Homogenous density, inner, upper chest wall C6-T26
Homogenous opacification of lung/s
　Bilateral C6-T10
　Unilateral C6-T11
Hyaline membrane disease, complications C6-T8
Hydronephrosis C15-T7
Hyperinflation C6-T13
Hyperlucent thorax C6-T14
Hypoaeration, hypoinflation C6-T15
Hypoplasia, pulmonary
　Associated with C6-T22
　Unilateral C6-T21
Interstitial emphysema C6-T12
Intra-abdominal calcifications C9-T23
Intraperitoneal calcifications C14-T3
Jaundice, obstructive C10-T4, C11-T1
Low bowel obstruction C9-T20
Lucencies, total body opacification C15-T5
Lung disease C6-T2
Meconium plug syndrome C9-T19
Microcolon of disuse C9-T22
Nephrogram C15-T6

Obstruction
    Gastric outlet C9-T16
    Intestinal C9-T9-T11
        High C9-T12
    Jaundice C11-T1
    Low bowel C9-T20
    Urinary bladder C15-T9
Opacification of hemithorax C6-T11
    Mediastinal displacement, contralateral side C6-T24
Osteolytic lesion C1-T13
Paralytic ileus C9-T5
Parenchymal disease C6-T16
Patchy alveolar infiltrations, asymmetric C6-T17
Perforation, hollow viscus C9-T24
Perirenal urinoma C15-T8
Platlet atelectasis C6-T20
Pleural effusion C6-T25
Pneumomediastinum C6-T12
Pneumoperitoneum C9-T25, C14-T2
Pneumothorax C6-T12
Portal vein, gas C9-T26
Pulmonary edema C8-T7
Pulmonary hemorrhage (a complication of…) C6-T9
Pulmonary hypoplsia C6-T22
Pulmonary veins or lymphatics, distended C8-T14
Pulmonary venous hypertrnsion C8-T6
Regurgitation, nasopharyngeal C9-T3
Renal mass, bilateral C15-T3, T4
Respiratory dystress
    Shifting of mediatinum C6-T23
Reticulo-nodular infiltrates C6-T6
Segmental atelectasis C6-T19
Soap-bubble appearance of intestine C9-T18
Soft-tissue edema C1-T16
Swallowing disorders C9-T2
Total body opacification C15-T5
Tracheo-esophageal fistula C6-T41, C9-T40
Unilateral hyperlucent thorax C6-T14
Urinary bladder outlet obstruction C15-T9
Urinoma, perirenal C15-T8

Shape C4-T3
Small, shallow cavity C4-T1
Oropharynx, mass, tumor C4-T52
Ossification
    Advanced, femoral head, premature C1-T12
    Center, fragmented, stippled C1-T20
    Defective, skull C3-T23
    Supernumerary centers C1-T21
Osteoarthropathy, hypertrophic C1-T69
Osteoblastic metastasis C1-T98
Osteoid formation, irregularities, zone of calcification C1-T32
Osteolysis, phalanges C1-T144
Osteolytic lesions of bone C1-T99
    Cervical spine C2-T15
    Expansile, primary tumor of bone C1-T96
    Ill defined, skull, multiple C3-T31
    Metaphysis, newborn C1-T13
    Vertebra/e C2-T14
    Punched-out, skull C3-T30
    Sternum C1-T109
Osteopenia/Osteoporosis
    Generalized C1-T77
    Localized C1-T78
    Vertebrae C2-T8
Osteosclerosis, bone dysplasia C1-T8
Osteosclerotic lesions, multiple C1-T82
Outflow obstruction, urinary bladder C15-T9, T59
Outlet obstruction
    Antral C9-T46
    Stomach C9-T16
    Urinary bladder, newborn C15-T9
Overlaping cranial sutures C3-T10
Overtubulation, long bones C1-T50

P
Pancreas
    Calcification C13-T4
    Mass C13-T1
        Tail region C13-T2
    Pseudocyst C13-T3

Papillary necrosis, kidney C15-T33
Paradoxical movement of diaphragm C7-T27
Paralytic ileus C9-T83
    Newborn C9-T5
Paramedial, midline calcification/s of skull C3-T46
Paranasal sinuses
    Destruction C4-T44
    Hypoplasia C4-T37
    Large C4-T38
    Mass C4-T45
        Opacification C4-T39
        With bone destruction C4-T43, T44
    Underdeveloped C4-T36
Paraspinal, soft-tissue mass C2-T50, C17-T3
Parathyroid gland, large C5-T3
Parenchyma (See also Lung and Parenchyma)
    Bronchiectasis C6-T87
    Calcification
        Bilateral C6-T102
        Solitary C6-T103
    Cavitation formation C6-T88
    Congestion, reticular pattern C6-T79
    Cyst C6-T90
        Multiple
            Bilateral C6-T92
            Unilateral C6-T91
            With fluid level C6-T94
        Solitary, with or without fluid level C6-T93
    Cyst-like structure C6-T18
    Densities
        Linear C6-T78
        Wedge-shaped C6-T78
    Edema, pulmonary C6-T80, T81
        Unilateral C6-T82
    Hemorrhage C6-T83
    Honeycomb pattern C6-T86
    Hyperinflation, hyperaeration C6-T57
        Unilateral C6-T58
    Hyperlucent, hemithorax, children C6-T105
    Hypoinflation

Left-to-right shunt at the level of the main pulmonary artery (Trunk) C8-T49
Main segment (Trunk)
    Aortic knob, bulge C8-T37
    Concave C8-T46
    Convex C8-T47
    Flat C8-T45
    Prominent C8-T48
Cavitary C6-T88
Consolidation, pleural effusion and rib rerefication C6-T111
Cyst
    Bilateral or multiple C6-T92
    With fluid levels C6-T94
Cyst-like structures C6-T90
    Unilateral C6-T91
Edema C8-T7, T55, T56
Hemorrhage
    Newborn C6-T9
    Older infants C6-T83
Hypoplasia
    Associated with…C6-T22
    Unilateral, newborn C6-T21
Infarction C6-T84
Interstitial fibrosis C6-T85
Lesion, cavitation formation C6-T88
Multiple, mass or nodule C6-T88
Pathology, with or without pleural effusion C6-T108
Pneumatocele C6-T89
Psedotumor C6-T101
Round lesion in leukemic patient C6-T69
Unequal pulmonary blood flow C8-T51
Vascular
    Abnormal pattern C8-T52
    Congestion or edema C8-T53, T55
    Venous hypertension C8-T6
Vascularity
    Cyanosis
    Arterial
        Decreased C8-T13, T16
        Increased C8-T12, T15

Lethal, neonatal C1-T1
Non-lethal C1-T5
Short rib C1-T118
Short sacro-iliac notch C1-T158
Shunt
    Left-to-right shunt at the level of the main pulmonary artery C8-T49
    Ventriculo-peritoneal, complications C3-T17
Sign
    Wimberger C1-T36
Single
    Bone lesion/s C1-T83
    Exostosis C1-T101, T102
    Platyspondyly C2-T11
    Pulmonary nodule C6-T96
Sinus wall destruction C4-T43, T44
Sinusitis
    Chronic C4-T41
    Maxillary with nasal drainage C4-T42
Skeletal bone tumors, benign, malignant C1-T94-T97
Skull, (see also Cranium)
    Asymmetry C3-T3
    Base, hypoplasia C3-T32
    Basilar invagination C3-T33
    Birth trauma C3-T55
    Bony changes around sella turcica C3-T43
    Calcification C3-T4
        Around sella turcica C3-T48
        Basal ganglia C3-T49
        Cerebral falx C3-T47
        Intracranial mass C3-T44, T50
        Midline and paramedial C3-T46
        Multiple C3-T45
        Supra- or infra-tentorial C3-T51
    Cloverleaf skull C3-T13
    Complications of fracture C3-T56
    Convolutional markings
        Decreased C3-T27
        Increased C3-T26
    Craniolacunia C3-T25
    Craniosynostosis C3-T11

Posterior cranial fossa
    Large C3-T34
    Small C3-T35
Separation of sutures C3-T7
Short base C3-T32
Small
    Anterior fontanel C3-T15
    Sella turcica C3-T39
    Shallow posterior fossa C3-T35
    Skull C3-T2
Space occupying lesion
    Infratentorial C3-T53
    Supratentorial C3-T52
Synostosis C3-T11
Thick
    Base C3-T21
    Bone/s C3-T19
    Localized C3-T20
Thining
    Generalized C3-T24
    Localized C3-T29
Trigonocephaly C3-T12
Tumor metastazing outside the CNS C3-T54
Unilateral expansion C3-T5
Ventriculo-peritoneal shunt, complications C3-T17
Wide dorsum sella C3-T41
Wide sutures C3-T7, T8, T18
Wormian bones, increased number C3-T9
Slender
    Clavicle C1-T114
    Rib C1-T122
Slipped epiphysis, femoral head C1-T163
Small
    Acetabular angle C1-T155
    Anterior fontanel C3-T15
    Epipihysis/es C1-T19
    Heart, microcardia C8-T34
    Kidney
        Bilateral C15-T19
        Unilateral C15-T20

Solitary
    Calcification, lung C6-T103
    Cyst, lung, with or without air-fluid level C6-T93
    Rib lesion C1-T125
Space joint
    Narrow C1-T179
    Wide C1-T178
Space occupying lesion
    Infratentorial C3-T53
    Intraperitoneal C14-T5
    Supratentorial C3-T52
    Urinary bladder C15-T65
Space, retrorectal, large C9-T87
Spine, (See also Vertebral)
    Cervical kyphosis C2-T35
    Increased lordosis C2-T42
    Kyphosis C2-40
    Scoliosis C2-T138-T40
        Complications after repair C2-T43
    Torticolis C2-T37
Splenic calcification C12-T4
Splenomegaly C12-T1
Splitting, cortex C1-T53
Spoge, kidney, medullary C15-T30
Stenosis
    Tracheal lumen C6-T39, T40
    Ureterovesical junction C15-T53
Step deformation, vertebrae C2-T7
Sternum
    Anomalies C1-T105
    Bone fusion C1-T105
    Osteolytic lesion C1-T109
    Pectus carinatum C1-T108
    Pectus excavatum C1-T107
    Premature segmental fusion C1-T106
Stiff, small bowel loops C9-T62
Stippled epiphysis C1-T20
Stomach
    Antral outlet obstruction C9-T46
    Displaced C9-T50

Toxic megacolon C9-T81
Trabecular pattern, coarse, bone C1-T80
Trabeculated urinary bladder wall C15-T63
Trachea, mass between C7-T9
Tracheal
    Bowing C6-T43
    Bronchus C6-T48
    Calcifications C6-T49
    Displacement C6-T46, C7-T9
    Isomerism C6-T51
    Narrowing C6-T39, T40
        Long segment C6-T45
        Short segment C6-T44
    Obstruction C6-T42
    Stenosis or narrowing C6-T39, T40, T44, T45
    Tracheal bronchus is associated with C6-T48
    Tracheo(broncho)megaly C6-T47
Tracheal bronchus is associated with…C6-T48
Tracheo(broncho)megaly C6-T47
Tracheoesophageal
        Communication C6-T41, C9-T40
Transverse, band, radiolucent metaphysis C1-T33
Trigonocephaly C3-T12
Triradiate acetabulum C1-T157
Tubulation, under-, long bones C1-T49
Tumor
    Bone, primary C1-T94-T97
    Broncho-parenchymal C6-T100
    Intrathoracic C6-T95
    Jaw C4-T23
    Metaztazing outside the CNS C3-T54
    Pharynx C4-T52
    Stomach C9-T47
    Vertebra, posterior arch C2-T32
Typhlitis C9-T74

U
Ulcer
    Duodenum C9-T53
    Esophagus C9-T33

Dorsum sella turcica C3-T41
Duodenal loop C9-T58
Esophagus C9-T36
Growth plate, generalized C1-T30
    Localized C1-T29
    Premature closure C1-T31
Joint space C1-T178
Meta-diaphyseal C1-T42
Ribs C1-T123
Symphysis pubis C1-T159
Widening
    Intervertebral disc space C2-T44
    Mediastinum
        Bilateral C7-T10
        Superior C7-T12
        Unilateral C7-T11
    Paraspinal soft-tissue C17-T3
    Soft-tissue of neck C5-T4
Wimberger metaphyseal sign C1-T36
Wings, butterfly C8-T56
Wormian bones of skull, increased number C3-T9

Z
Zone of provizional calcification, osteoid formation, irregularities C1-T32

978-0-595-34446-8
0-595-34446-1

www.ingramcontent.com/pod-product-compliance
Lightning Source LLC
Chambersburg PA
CBHW030939180526
45163CB00002B/628